THE FIVE ELEMENTS of
ACUPUNCTURE and CHINESE MASSAGE

THE FIVE ELEMENTS OF ACUPUNCTURE AND CHINESE MASSAGE

*A concise introductory work to the
theory and technique of Acupuncture*

by

DENIS LAWSON-WOOD, F.Ac.A.
&
JOYCE LAWSON-WOOD

HEALTH SCIENCE PRESS
Denington Estate, Wellingborough
Northamptonshire

First published 1965
Second Impression 1966
Second Edition,
completely revised and reset,
March 1973

ISBN 0 85032 106 9

Typeset by Specialised Offset Services, Liverpool
and printed by Straker Brothers Ltd., Whitstable

Contents

Preface

At least one of the goals expressed in the first edition of *Chinese System of Healing* (Health Science Press, 1959) has been to an appreciable extent achieved — namely, that of stimulating wide interest in Chinese acupuncture among English-speaking people.

When the book, the first in the English language to be published on the subject, appeared in 1959 only a relative handful had heard of Chinese acupuncture. To-day, six years later, extensive publicity through press, radio and television, has so reversed the situation that now it is only the few who have not yet heard about this Far-Eastern therapy. We feel some satisfaction, therefore, in having taken such an early part in paving the way for other authors who, coming later, will not have had to experience many of the difficulties inevitably associated with pioneering work.

We acknowledge with gratitude the many letters of criticism, constructive suggestions, and appreciation from practitioners who have successfully applied acupuncture when their only text was a copy of the first edition — which text was intended as introductory only to a very limited aspect of but one branch of Far-Oriental medicine.

New Material
This present work contains much material from the first

book, but so re-arranged, amplified, brought up-to-date, and new material added that it must now be considered as a new work rather than as a second edition. The new material has been in the main adapted from notes of many lectures given by us to students of acupuncture during these last few years.*

It is also gratifying to see our hope gradually attaining fulfilment, in that acupuncture and Chinese massage is becoming available ever more widely to the public through individual practitioners, groups and associations of healers whose knowledge, experience, skill, sincerity of purpose and professional code are at the highest level. The majority of these practitioners are, like ourselves, non-registered, non-medical health practitioners practising in conformity with naturopathic principles.

We would point out that a training in current Western (allopathic) medicine, far from being the essential preliminary that some would have the public believe, is far more likely to be a serious hindrance to sound acupuncture: for the simple reason that the basic medicine philosophies of East and West are poles apart. There are some who assert that before being allowed by law to practise acupuncture there should first be a qualification and registration as a doctor of medicine. Such critics show lamentable ignorance of Far-Eastern medicine philosophy; and, in our view, any practitioner expressing such 'closed shop' restriction should himself not pretend to practise traditional acupuncture.

As, for example, in the field of sport, it would be absurd to require knowledge and skill in table tennis or football *in order to play* cricket: so too in the therapeutic field it appears absurd to require knowledge of one set of rules *in*

---

* e.g. Training courses given under the auspices of the Acupuncture Association, the British College of Acupuncture, etc., as well as numerous privately arranged small groups and classes.

order to observe a different set. One can appreciate, in sport, that by applying inappropriate rules and skills, an amusing even exciting game might result but it would not be cricket. Likewise inappropriate rules might result in a valid therapy, perhaps a dangerous therapy, but it would not be Chinese acupuncture.

When, however, it is practised in accordance with the appropriate medicine-philosophical orientation and knowledge, traditional acupuncture is a valid therapy and it is not dangerous. *It can be dangerous only when practised by someone so conditioned in an inappropriate discipline that his mind has not the flexibility so necessary to the understanding of Far-Eastern philosophy and basic principles of the art and science of healing.*

Art of Prevention

The essential art is that of foreseeing and preventing rather than treating sickness after it has become manifested in painful or distressing bodily and mental symptoms. In the West the average practitioner's first contact with the patient does not generally occur until after symptoms have made their appearance: thus the Western healer's first task will, of necessity, be that of restoring a sick person to a state of health, rather than maintaining the good health of a healthy person.

Since it is written for the Westerner this work must be concerned with Western conditions. Even though some data herein may be of use to the average intelligent person to use his fingers as massage instruments to cope with symptoms that have already made their appearance, it must be emphasized that *at no time are symptoms to be suppressed.* Always one aims to remove causes at a deep level. The ONLY justification for palliative measures is that of expediency, *to make curative treatment possible.* The pure Hahnemannian homoeopath will understand this:

for his medicine philosophy runs closely parallel to that of his Far-Eastern colleague.

We do not herein take sides in the allopathic/ homoeopathic controversy — we do not assert that one is right, the other wrong. We do however assert that they are different and opposed, therefore not to be mixed.

As he cannot go in two opposite directions at one and the same time, each practitioner has to choose for himself which path to follow — East or West. Each will, of course, choose the path which (according to his interpretation of the sign-post) offers optimum probability of leading to the one and only ultimate valid therapy — 'that which heals the patient'.

D.L.-W. & J.L.-W. 1965.
TUNBRIDGE WELLS

1.

Yang and Yin

YANG and YIN are the only two Chinese words we shall be constantly using. It is, therefore of first importance that we explain as clearly as we are able what notions are embodied in these two terms. Unless a student gets a thorough grasp of the philosophic concepts of YANG and YIN he cannot hope to make any real headway in the art and science of acupuncture-point therapy.

If one seeks to practise acupuncture without knowing the basic philosophy there is the danger of becoming a mere technician – that is to say, treating symptoms by formulae and reference to a repertory in the manner of what the Chinese call the 'inferior doctor'. All the same, as a technician, one might well become proficient and score a high percentage of good results, but that is not the 'high art' we aim to master.

Far-Eastern Science
Just because the label 'philosophy' is used there is no need to jump to the conclusion that the subject is therefore difficult. Far from it. We believe the concepts involved are extremely simple. That so many people experience difficulty with philosophy is not because the subject itself is difficult, but rather because of the way in which the notions are presented. We will do what we can to present in simple non-technical terms a broad general picture of

the relevant Far Eastern notions of cosmogeny. The doctrine of how this universe and everything in it came into being in the first place, and then became what it now appears is *the foundation teaching* upon which all Far-Eastern Science (including acupuncture) is built.

From the standpoint of Western science, Far-Eastern science may appear 'unscientific' and altogether too philosophical or even religious. Nevertheless if once the basic premises are clearly stated, explained, and understood, it will be found that the whole system is superbly logical — to satisfy even the most rigid logician.

A precise and brief formulation of the Basic Premise (One Law) and twelve axiomatic propositions, is attributed to FU HSI, the legendary Emperor who, according to various authorities is supposed to have lived between 8000 and 5000 years ago. This One Law and Twelve Propositions provide us with the essential data of the *laws of nature governing the universe.* These laws are absolute and inviolable; no creature, thing, or circumstance can escape them.

FU HSI's One Law states:

'The universe represents the interplay of the two activities Yang and Yin, and their vicissitudes.'

The twelve propositions go on to elaborate this, giving us carefully ordered detail. Before listing these propositions we give these few notes, to explain something of what they tell us. The *first* proposition tells us WHAT made the universe, and OF WHAT it is made. The *second* tells us HOW it happened; it informs us that 'creation' is none other than the coming into being of a bi-polar energy (or more simply, of bi-polarity). The *third* concerns the nature of the two poles. *Fourthly* we are told of what substance Beings and Phenomena are made. Then, fifth, we are enlightened concerning the nature of Beings and Phenomena. The *sixth* proposition tells us of the governing relationship of attraction between the two poles. The *seventh* gives us the first basis of Relativity, namely that both poles always co-exist: and, in the *eighth*, we learn that nothing but polar activity exists. Then, in the *ninth*, we are informed concerning the strength of the attraction of one pole for its opposite. The *tenth*, on the other hand, tells us of the strength of the repulsion of a pole for its similar. In the last two propositions we learn about Time and Space: the *eleventh* tells us how continuity happens; or, about the nature of Time, Periodicity, Rhythm, etc., and, finally in the *twelfth* proposition, the nature of Space, Form, or relative positions of polar energy charges.

FU HSI's formulation is more than a story of Creation it is also a 'Story of Continuum'.

It would be well for the serious student to commit the One Law and twelve axiomatic propositions to memory. This need not be an intolerable burden — memorizing will be found to take place more or less automatically and with little effort, simply by re-reading and reflecting upon what is read.

The One Law
The Universe represents the interplay of the two activities YANG and YIN, and their vicissitudes.

Twelve Axiomatic Propositions
1. That which produces and composes the Universe is TAO, Inner Nature. (Also may be translated: Zero, Nothing or Universe-AEther.)
2. Inner Nature (Zero) polarizes itself: one pole becomes charged with Yang activity, the other with Yin activity.
3. Yang and Yin are opposites.
4. Beings and Phenomena in the Universe are multiple and complex aggregates of Universe-AEther charged

with Yang and Yin in all proportions.

5. Beings and Phenomena are divers dynamic equilibra: nothing in the universe is stable or finished; all is in unceasing motion, because polarization, the South of Being, is without beginning and without end.

6. Yang and Yin attract one another.

7. Nothing is wholly Yin nor wholly Yang. Yin and Yang are characterized only relatively: all is Yin and Yang aggregate.

8. Nothing is neutral. Polarization is ceaseless and universal.

9. The force of attraction between two beings is a function of the difference between their charges of opposite activities (expressed in mathematical symbols $A = f(x-y)$.)

10. Like activities repel one another. The repulsion between two beings of the same polarity is the greater the closer their similarity.

11. Yin produces Yang: Yang produces Yin.

12. All beings are charged: Yang interiorly, Yin exteriorly.

A thorough understanding of Yang and Yin is not merely a basic requisite for the understanding of acupuncture – there is no department of human interest where the principles of the working of Yang and Yin do not apply. In these principles we have a key to unlock the door to almost any mystery, or to point the way to the solution of almost any problem in any and every field of human thought, activity and endeavour.

If, for example, you happen to be interested in astronomy you will be able to offer a logically valid explanation of the fact that the heavenly bodies have an elliptical orbit. Modern Western science has not answered that one. Should you be interested in one of the most recent of all human activities, space travel, you would be able to forsee problems that sooner or later *will* arise in outer space: and you could tackle and solve them *before* a disaster brings them to notice.

We must now spend a little time examining FU HSI's formulations in greater detail.

We have designedly used the expression 'WHAT made the Universe?' rather than 'WHO made it?', because already, thousands of years ago in the Far East the sages appear to have arrived at the notion of the Creator as a *mathematical abstraction*, rather than the conception of a Person of exalted dimensions and peculiar characteristics.

Summary of Creation

The Chinese 'creation story' is summarized in the TAO TEH CHING, Chapter XLII, in these words:

'Tao gave birth to the One: the One gave birth successively to two things, three things, up to ten thousand. These ten thousand creatures cannot turn their backs to the shade without having the sun on their bellies, and it is upon this blending of the breaths that their harmony depends'*

We can say the same thing in another way: Tao, the Nothing (Absolute ZERO) became something by the primary act of asserting itself, and, in thus becoming, polarized itself into Yang and Yin.

Although assertion comes first, it implies the possibility of negation. We have thus the apparently paradoxical situation of Positive and Negative (Plus and Minus) happening *together* though Plus happens first!

We can think of this primary act of self-assertion (Zero becoming something) as a sort of 'focusing', 'organizing', creating a limitation, condensing to a point, etc. At the very instant of becoming something, *that something can become nothing*. Movement in one direction implies the

* Arthur Waley's translation.

possibility of movement in the opposite direction. This always applies. Let us take the simple example of *filling* a bowl with rice. When filled the bowl has *actual fullness* (of rice) *and a potential emptiness.*

Every organization can be disorganized;

Every focusing to a centre can be dispersed to a periphery;

Every 'living' implies 'dying';

Every birth implies death.

YANG and YIN (Plus and Minus) represent complements in the sense that one cannot exist without the other – each implies the other. At the same time the Plus and Minus can be viewed as antagonists: for the 'pull' or 'urge' of of each is the opposite direction to the other.

Yang and Yin – Cosmic Forces

These two urges or forces which operate throughout the entire cosmos were given the names YANG and YIN. These are the urges *to become something* (Yang) and *to return to nothing* (Yin).

Out of the primary act of polarization *primary matter* happens, i.e., 'The three things'; Essence, Movement, Form. From primary matter all things develop. In this context the expression 'the ten thousand things' simply means 'everything'.

From primary matter there came about successively the condensation of (or separation out into) general dense terrestrial matter; and the primary Elements. From these first *general* matters came the individual matters, things and organizations by process of individualization through combination of various proportions. Each and every individual (or special combination) resolves itself ultimately to a *manifestation* of bi-polar energy, of Yang and Yin. Where there is one pole there too *must* be the other. It cannot be otherwise.

The continued existence or harmony of any individual thing, creature, phenomenon, or circumstance, depends upon the maintaining of the relative proportions of Yang and Yin appropriate to that individual.

This unitary bi-polar energy is the Substance out of which everything is made. According to the degree, quality, manner of 'holding together', it may appear as solid, liquid, gaseous, radiant, etc.

The student will readily appreciate that, if focusing to a point were continued *unimpeded* there would come about a disappearance into the Centre. Therefore unless we have at the same time as a movement inwards towards centre a counter-balancing effort from the centre outwards, there would still be nothing real. Likewise, of course, if the effort from centre to periphery were continued unimpeded, there would be dispersion to nothing. The two forces must co-exist and dynamically balance one another for something to exist.

Matter as Energy

The notion that 'solid matter' is not 'solid', but is none other than a special appearance or form of energy is not altogether foreign to Westerners. Modern Western scientists seem to be coming round to the idea that everything and every appearance in this world is only 'energy' behaving in some special way. Modern Western scientists also seem to agree that ultimately all is reducible to one primary Energy. Sir James Jeans, F.R.S., states that the substance of this universe is empty space welded on to empty time. A poetic way of saying that the substance of this world is a manifestation of Nothing: or 'Zero realized as Something'.*

The 'picture' Jeans seems to favour is the picture

* *The Mysterious Universe*, Cambridge, 1930.

provided by the wave-mechanics of *de Broglie and Schrödinger*. He, however, informs us that 'the essential fact is simply that *all the* pictures which science now draws of nature, and which alone seem capable of according with observational fact, are mathematical pictures'.

He also tells us that modern scientists are finding, in a whole torrent of surprising new knowledge, that appearances in this world are more fully, more naturally, and more clearly explained by the mathematical way, in terms of mathematical concepts.

Answering certain objections, Jeans tell us that 'it would of course have proved nothing, if nature had merely been found to act in accordance with the concepts of applied mathematics, for the concepts of applied mathematics have been specially and deliberately designed by man to fit the workings of nature.'

But when it comes to the more intricate concepts of pure mathematics he writes that it can hardly be disputed that *nature and our conscious mathematical minds work according to the same Laws.* He seems to consider there is sufficient justification for thinking of the designer of the universe as a mathematician; and the universe can best be pictured as consisting of pure thought of a mathematical thinker or universal mind.

Universe of Pure Thought

The 'ideas' of the 'mathematical thinker' are referred to in the TAO TEH CHING as the 'secret essences' or 'simple essences'.

'This concept of the universe as a world of pure thought throws new light on many of the situations we have encountered in our survey of modern physics. We can see how the ether, in which all the events of the universe take place, could reduce to a mathematical abstraction, and become as abstract as mathematical parallels of latitude and meridians of longitude. We can also see why *energy, the fundamental entity of the universe*, had again to be treated as a mathematical abstraction – the constant of integration of a differential equation.'*

A hundred-and-sixty years ago a German naturalist, Lorenz Oken, wrote: 'Nature is the manifestation of mathematical ideas.'†

Lorenz Oken has received too little attention up to the present day; it is our considered opinion that his often derided notions may yet form the basis for advanced Western modern science, for his theories run closely parallel to traditional scientific thought of many Far Eastern sages of thousands of years ago.

The one bi-polar energy not only manifests as various solids, liquids, gases, etc., as the 'building units' but it must also be considered as activating the various conglomerations and complex aggregates. If we look upon this one bi-polar energy as having ever so many *levels* of manifestation, from the most subtle invisible to the coarsest and grossest visible, we see that each level in some way could be expected, to some degree, to influence at least the levels immediately above and below. Actually what does appear to happen is that an *event on one level affects an analagous or corresponding event on every other level.*

If we wish to bring about a change of appearance or change of activity manifestation on one or more particular levels we seek the level having the strongest overriding influence that is accessible to us. The level of energy manifestation which has, as far as the health and well-being in mind and body of a human being is concerned, dominant or controlling influence will be the level the

* Jeans, op. cit. Italics are ours.
† *Elements of Physiophilosophy.*

therapist aims to manipulate. We refer to the level having the strongest influence over all the others as the *deepest level*. Changes brought about at the deepest level will bring about *related* changes in the other levels.

Western therapy in general seems directed towards influencing energy at 'blood' or at 'nerve-energy' level; at visible cell and tissue level; or at some microscopic level. All these levels just mentioned are relatively superficial levels for overriding control purposes.

Far-Oriental therapy considers a circulation of energy on an extremely subtle sub-microscopic level. We say sub-microscopic with some reservation, for researches at present being carried out point to the possibility of instrumental revelation of a cell formation and of a circulation, in the human body, which has hitherto not been noticed.*

Life Force

According to Far-Eastern teaching there is a subtle energy manifestation circulating in the viscera, in the flesh, and ultimately permeating every living cell and tissue. The name given to *this* energy form, at this particular level, is translated as Life Force (Vital Force, Vital Energy, etc). We sometimes simply call it Energy.

This Energy is considered as having clearly distinct and established pathways. definite direction of flow, characteristic behaviour, etc., quite as definite as any other circulation on other levels, such as blood and vascular system.

Tradition has it that there are Inner, Outer, and Connecting circulations of Life Force. The principal Inner circulation is that which flows through and unites the inner organs; the Outer circulation, or the peripheral

* *On the Kyungrak System – The Scientific, material Bases of Acupuncture*, thesis by Professor Kim Bongham, November 1963, Pyongyang, North Korea.

circulation, occurs just below the skin surface.

Energy on or near the surface can be directly contacted and influenced by manipulation or some form of treatment. The Inner circulation, and the circulations linking Inner and Outer, not being directly accessible is influenced through surface points having appropriate links with the internal. The superficial or peripheral channels of Vital Energy together comprise the *Circulation System* known as *the Meridian Circulation.* The Energy pathways or meridians have been traditionally mapped out, and the various control or 'key' points on these meridians are well established. These points. at which Life Force can be effectively and predictably controlled are known as *Acupuncture Points.*

They have been called acupuncture points because the chief traditional method of influence is by means of needle insertion and manipulation of the needle.

One is not limited to use of a needle at the points – there are several alternative ways of manipulating the Life Energy *with equal effectiveness.* The two principal alternatives being *Massage* and Cauterization (Moxa = Burning Herb).

Some of the acupuncture points are used to control Surface Energy directly; some to influence indirectly the inner Core Energy; some to influence the intermediate circulations which link Inner and Outer, or which constitute Energy 'reserves'.

We shall be returning to these Meridians and Organs later on: we must now continue with the consideration of the more general nature and behaviour of Yang and Yin. The notion 'dynamic equilibra' now calls for attention.

Life Process, or more appropriately Existence Process, is not simply a series of static conditions, but complexes of processes occurring as rhythmic creations of tensions and relaxations of these tensions. This can also be described as 'polarising' followed by 'de-polarizing': or building up a 'charge' followed by a 'discharge' of energy: activity and repose.

The stimulation of one pole evokes its opposite, creating a tension which, through movement, resolves itself. In its turn *movement polarizes*, creating new tension for resolution, and so on unceasingly throughout Space-Time.

2.

Periodicity and Rhythm

Periodicity or Rhythm is everywhere to be observed in nature. Some processes are so rapid that we are not able to become aware of them through our senses; likewise some processes are too slow for us to register. As a matter of expediency we tend to look upon the very slow processes as if they were static – but here static only means relatively so. In between the two extremes there are numberless cognizable processes on many levels. They ALL conform to the one fundamental process pattern, the Polarity pattern.

Every cosmic system and process has its microscopic counterpart in man. The nature of Change (life, existence) is PROCESS and NOT catastrophe.

Everything that exists has a beginning or stage of *minimum existence*, and a stage of maturity or *maximum existence*. The transition from minimum to maximum, and maximum to minimum represents the fundamental rhythm or cycle in nature.

Two examples of this rhythm are illustrated in the rather simplified instance of the life cycle of a plant, and the yearly cycle in a tree (whose life-cycle may extend over many years). (*see DIAGRAMS*)

In these instances of cycles we have represented them diagramatically as circular, but, we feel, they should be visualized rather more in the nature of spirals than flat closed circles.

DIAGRAMMATIC REPRESENTATION OF A NATURAL CYCLE: PLANT GROWTH

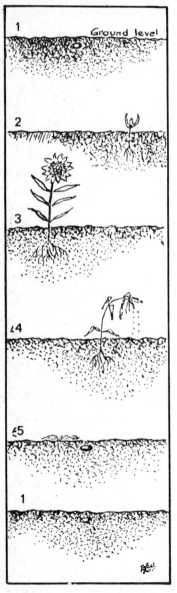

STAGE 1.
> Below the ground a seed or plant in a state of minimum; just prior to the first stirrings into activity.

STAGE 2.
> In SPRING the young shoot shows above ground and strives upwards towards light, air, etc. GROWTH towards maturity.

STAGE 3.
> SUMMER or MATURITY. The plan is shewn with its seed-containing blossom at its maximum.

STAGE 4.
> Late Summer, DECREASE or withdrawal of life begins when the seed is ripe for gathering or falls to the ground.

STAGE 5.
> AUTUMN the season of gathering, stirring, or the seed becomes buried. This is the stage of BALANCE.

As Stage 1 Finally in WINTER once more the minimum; the new seed lies dormant ready for the coming spring when the cycle begins again and fulfils itself anew. This is known as the stage of the power of EMPTINESS.

*DIAGRAMMATIC REPRESENTATION OF THE
YEARLY RHYTHM OF A TREE*

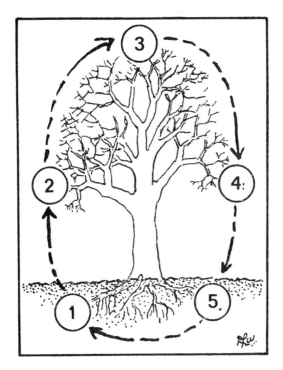

1. in WINTER the sap lies relatively dormant in the roots.
2. in SPRING the sap level rises.
3. and reaches the outer limits in SUMMER.
4. With the formation of mature fruit in LATE SUMMER the receding or DECREASE begins.
5. Fruit and leaves fall in AUTUMN: the sap level recedes below ground to lie in store for the cycle to begin once more at the proper time.

In the rising and falling of the sap, it is not that the flow of sap changes from a flow upwards to a flow downwards, but rather that the height to which the ever upward-flowing sap reaches recedes or rises.

Cyclic Processes

The more complex the form of life, the more cyclic processes are to be found taking place, at different speeds, different cycle durations, on various levels, all interweaving, intermingling, influencing each other, etc. Whether a cycle completes itself in a few moments, hours, days, months or years, the ancients considered the process stages all to conform to a basic pattern. We shall go into this more deeply later on in the Five Elements Doctrine. The basic notion to grasp here is that of Polarization of a Unitary Force into Positive and Negative poles: first there is a predominance of Positive moving outwards from minimum to maximum positive, then decrease of positive (increase of negative) leading to predominance of negative in the return movement to minimum.

We make no apologies for the time now being spent on this aspect: it should prove to be time well spent, in order to get a deep 'organismic feel' of the bi-polar orientation.

Formation and Movement

We illustrate these ideas further with a quick reference to the formation and movement of heavenly bodies. This is highly significant in that according to the teaching that man is a microcosm, we can learn a great deal about our own organs, functions, etc., through observation of cosmic happenings.

It is supposed that 'In the Beginning' there was a tensioning to a point of inequality in the undifferentiated AEther of Space, creating a focal point of SUCTION, or condensation to a centre, together with Rotation. Thus there was a centripetal urge, an urge outwards from centre to periphery.

In this way a central Core, or Sun, is formed, which becomes surrounded by a series of hollow (concentric) globes — in layers somewhat like the skin and layers of an onion. The rotating hollow globes condense into planetary Rings which rotate with the centre. Saturn's rings are an instance of satellite formation arrested at the ring stage. The planetary rings further condense to form spherical planetary bodies.

Sun and Planet are related polarwise to each other. The planet is both drawn towards the Sun by centripetal action, and repelled away from the Sun by centrifugal action. *The planet itself is bi-polar.*

It is a peculiarity of planetary bodies that they change their polarity predominance by their own power. We quote in full two paragraphs from Oken's *Elements of Physiophilosophy*, as this seems to accord with traditional far-eastern cosmogeny:

par. 234. The circumvolution of the planets around the sun is a *polar* process of *attraction* and *repulsion*, by virtue of the primary law in the solar system, by virtue of the light. The planet then can only be repelled in the neighbourhood of the sun from the sun, when it has the *same* solar pole in itself, when it has become positive; and can only attract it at a distance from the sun, when it has received the opposite pole to the sun, or has become negative.

par. 235. This is only conceivable in that the planet, while it draws nearer to the sun, extinguishes in itself by its *own* power the negative pole, and produces on the contrary the positive pole, or becomes a sun: and that, as it removes itself from the sun, it again extinguishes the positive solar pole, and generates the negative planetary pole within itself. This substantial production of alternating poles upon the planet takes place through the diversity of its surface as water and land, through the oblique position of its axis, whereby summer and winter are produced, through the processes, or through the life that is upon it, through the processes of decomposition and combination effected by water, through the revival and death of vegetation, even the white colour of snow. The planet discharges its pole in the neighbourhood of the sun, like a cork pellet, and reloads of itself at a distance from the sun; and thus oscillates to and fro, like the hammer in an electric bell. The course of the planets takes place with the greatest ease. It is everywhere no force of weight, of impulse, but of the easiest self-motion. The planet revolves by its own force to and from the sun, like the blood circulates to and from the heart.

(*Elements of Physiophilosophy*. English translation 1847).

We shall be examining the circulation of the blood as a polar process in a few moments. The essential point to grasp now is that each planetary manifestation has, *within itself*, both Plus and Minus poles. First the one pole predominates then the other. This is the basic pattern which we shall later on see carried out in the meridians' energy.

Negative and Positive Urges

Provided that the bi-polar Energy undergoes the natural rhythmic changes at the proper times at the proper speeds, strengths, etc., the Event, Being, or Circumstance, System or Organization remains constant and we say that it is living in health. The balance of Negative and Postitive Urges has to be maintained within limits appropriate to the particular manifestation.

We return, momentarily, to our example of the TREE and the SAP. The tree sap, or *life-blood of the tree*, is considered as a planetary body related polarwise to Earth Centre. The limit of closeness to the centre is marked by the tops of the roots: and the furthermost limit is marked by the extremities of the outer twigs. There is a seasonal rhythmic change of polarity; the sap level rises and recedes in seasonal rhythm.

We should mention here than an *individual* tree is looked upon, NOT as a complete planet, but as *part* of a planet. The complete 'tree planet' is made up of all trees of that kind upon the whole earth surface, forming a broad ring (or double ring, one north and one south of the equator). The planetary 'ring-wave' travels round the earth with a tide-like motion.

PLANT LIFE, i.e., *all* plant life represents the totality of *internally moved* bodies: each individual member is *bound to one location on the earth surface.*

ANIMAL LIFE represents a different class of life, namely, Organic Bodies *moved throughout.* Each member, or individual animal, having its own centre, to which its own periphery is polar-wise related. In other words, these organic bodies have within themselves both SOLAR and PLANETARY manifestations. ANIMAL LIFE, being a higher, that is to say *more complete* form of life than plants, includes within itself the lower forms, functions and activities.

In this context 'lower' and 'higher' is not in any way intended to mean 'more' or 'less' ethical, moral, or any other worth, but simply more *complete.*

In animal life there are *vegetative* functions and processes side by side with *animal* functions and processes: but the lower functions are raised to a new level.

Plant Life represents a micro-planet. Earth and Plant (planet) together representing a micro-solar system. Animal Life represents a micro-solar system in each individual member.

Man not in Animal Class

AS REGARDS MAN, Man does *NOT* belong to the animal

class of life. We feel this to be highly important for us in acupuncture; so important indeed that we would like you to underline it heavily in red, and never, never forget it. *This distinction is of immense therapeutic significance*, for, quite apart from the new dignity thus accorded to man, we shall be able to appreciate the inadequacy of drug and other experiments carried out upon animals and then attempting to apply the results to man.

MAN BELONGS TO A SPECIAL CLASS OF LIFE AND THEREFORE REQUIRES A THERAPEUTIC APPROACH APPROPRIATE TO THAT CLASS.

As we see it, acupuncture does represent a possible therapeutic approach which is appropriate to man. We use the term 'acupuncture' in a very broad sense to represent the traditional Far-Eastern medicine philosophic approach.

Man embodies an additional characteristic which raises him to a higher *more complete* class than animal. Each individual human represents a MICRO-COSM, and has within himself all the lower manifestations, processes, functions, etc., raised to a new level, in addition to his own HUMAN CHARACTERISTIC.

This realization was, in Western culture, *first* formulated and published (*circa* 1921) by Alfred Korzybski. The Tibetan C-S-B Doctrine, however, long ago recognized man's unique status; it placed Inorganic life in the Badgan mode; Organic life, plant and animal, in the Schara mode; and MAN in the Chi mode. The Human characteristic is psychic, or symbol-forming, which gives him freedom of movement in Time.

We feel that it is only upon recognition of the Human characteristic that psycho-therapy will become adequate and progress: and, moreover, if the outcome of this book is no more than a deep conviction, on the part of the reader, of the true status and dignity of human beings, we shall be satisfied this work has not been in vain.

3.

Life Processes

We now give one or two examples to illustrate how some bodily processes are to be viewed when one has become polar-wise oriented in one's thinking. These examples will also serve to elucidate FU HSI's propositions.

There are several different kinds of movement in the human body (also occurring in animals) which will include the following: (i) Movement of a fluid, e.g., blood, chyle, lymph, etc., (ii) movement of contractile tissue, (iii) movement of a nerve impulse, (iv) movement of air, as in respiration, (v) secretions, glandular and organ, etc.

(i) Circulation of a fluid is perhaps best exemplified in the circulation of blood. We are concerned to find an answer to the question 'Why does blood move?'

From the Yang/Yin 'polar' point of view the circulation of blood in the blood vessels, veins and arteries, is NOT a result of the mechanical pumping action of the heart, but is the result of Yang/Yin polar interplay. The pulsation of the heart is not a cause of circulation but rather is it a consequence thereof.

Extremes of Circulation
In this example we shall not unduly complicate matters by bringing into consideration the function of the liver. First let us locate the extremes or poles of the Circulation. What represents the Yang and the Yin?

The forces of Yang (combination) and Yin (separation)

are represented as oxygenation and de-oxygenation. Thus two extremes are lungs and capillaries. Blood in its *combined* condition is a nutrient fluid carrying oxygenated chyle. The Chinese considered blood to be made in the lungs. From their point of view they are correct since the *fully* combined condition is achieved in the lungs. Thus the lungs represent one of the extremes.

The other extreme of the circulation must be sought at the place where the condition is that of 'fully separated out'; that is to say, de-oxygenated non-chyliferous blood AND non-oxygenated uncoloured chyle. These will be found in the capillaries AND in the small intestine.

Yang attracts Yin: thus the chyle moves by polar tension between intestine and lung. Chyle at the small intestine has no oxygen and requires it. It moves therefore towards the oxygen pole, the lungs. In the capillaries the blood is de-oxygenated blood, separated out or empty-Yin. In its now 'empty' (Yin) condition it is attracted towards the Yang pole for re-oxygenation: it is also attracted towards the chyle in order to be re-charged with nutrient matter. The conductors of the fluids are the veins and lymphatic vessels. ON THEIR WAY to the lungs the non-oxygenated chyle and the de-oxydized or venous blood are mixed. This takes place in the heart.

In the words of the NEI CHING, 'The heart nourishes the blood'.

In the lungs, through oxydation, the chyle becomes coloured red, and nourishing or arterial blood is formed. The yangized blood is now of the same polarity as the lung, the Yang pole of the circulatory system. Like poles repel one another, the blood therefore is driven forcibly from the lungs and is attracted towards the Yin pole of the vascular system, namely the capillaries. On its way it passes through the heart. After reaching the capillaries and becoming separated out, the cycle is repeated.

Blood Flow Makes Heart Beat

It will be noted that un-oxygenated and oxygenated blood passes through the heart. This *flow* polarizes the muscles of the heart and rhythmically creates polar tension in the heart muscles, resulting in discharge of tension through muscle contraction, followed by momentary relaxation and renewed tension – the heart-beats. The heart forms the body's 'built-in clock'; or as some say, the heart is the body's pace-maker.

Though the heart may have some mechanical pumping action, this mechanical action is not the circulation's prime mover: bi-polar tension and discharge of tension causes circulation. Flow through the heart provides the necessary movement to polarize the heart muscles.

Blood *can* flow without the heart beating but the heart does not beat unless there is blood flow. A person may be revived even after the heart has stopped beating, so long as blood still flows, however feebly. Resuscitation techniques aim primarily to maintain or re-establish regular oxygenation or stimulation of the circulatory process, and only secondarily it stimulates the heart.

The heart-beat is, nevertheless, necessary to life, for the pulsation is felt throughout the organism and acts as the standard measure of periodicity for other cyclic processes.

(ii) Movement of contractile tissue as a manifestation of polar excitation, tension and discharge, can be exemplified in the contraction of striated muscle fibres. A muscle is to be considered as a bi-conical fibre with *unequal* cones. One cone is attached more or less directly to bone, at the muscle 'origin'; the other cone elongates into sinew or tendon of 'insertion'. Nerve stimulus induces polar excitation, building up a charge (or PD for discharge). The muscle Yang and Yin poles then attract one another. The poles move towards each other by contraction of the fibre. Discharge is followed by relaxation. In this case the excited energy is, in a sense, bound to the tissues and therefore *in moving* the bound energy moves the tissue to which it is bound.

(iii) In the case of nerve energy we also have a creation or activation of polar tension between the two ends of the nerve fibre. Here, however the tissue is not contractile, therefore in order that tension may be discharged (and the two ends of the fibre not being able to approximate) the 'charge' courses along the fibre as an energy impulse.

(iv) In the respiratory process, when we consider this as a flow of air, we need to look for the polar tensions as between air inside and air outside the lungs, with reference to their relative oxygen and carbon di-oxide ratios.

In-rush and out-flow of air constitutes movement which polarizes respiratory muscles. Here again we question whether the so-called respiratory muscles *cause* the in and out flow; or whether the respiratory muscles function should be considered as more regulatory than causative.

It is indisputable than an infant's *first* breath is NOT caused by action of the respiratory muscles, but by the expansion of the lungs due to the following sequence of happenings: The severance of the umbilical cord results in no further arterial blood arriving from the placenta (the 'foetal lung') through the umblical vein: the left heart is no longer stimulated and the foramen ovale collapses and is closed. All the blood enters the right side of the heart and, finding no way through into the ductus arteriosus it is driven forcibly into the lungs *which now expand*, thereby leaving empty space between the pulmonary vessels into which the air rushes.

The student will be amply repaid by devoting some time to careful re-consideration of the embryonic development of the circulation system, and noting the order in which specialized tissues appear.

Gastric Juice

(v) In organ and glandular secretions we can observe yet another manifestation of polar activity – creation of tension and its discharge. Let us consider here as our example the secretion of gastric juice – or, more widely, the phenomena of *hunger* and *thirst*.

Hunger and thirst are opposites in the sense that a person is *either* hungry *or* thirsty, but not both at one and the same time. There is ample justification for the recommendation made by dietitians that one should not drink with meals. Through the digestive process gastric juice is consumed. Secretion of gastric juice is an oxydizing process; gastric juice is *consumed by the food* – in other words, the *food acts as the de-oxydizing pole.* When there is a deficiency of de-oxydizing ailments the 'oxygenic tension' is heightened in the stomach to unpleasantness, producing a feeling which we call 'hunger'. This tension (hunger) can be described as either an excess of the oxydizing pole or as a deficiency of the de-oxydizing pole. Balance is restored by the introduction into the stomach of that which is deficient – or by a dispersal of that which is in excess.

Hunger, as a condition of 'emptiness' is a Yin condition. Yin also relates to *cold.* If body temperature is low, there is either excess Yin or deficiency of Yang. Eating something will appease the hunger feeling and raise body temperature.

On the other hand *thirst* indicates an excess of de-oxydation which may come about either from the de-oxydation process being too rapid (e.g., as from excess food) or from a deficiency of gastric juice secretion – resulting in a feeling of *dryness* or *heat*, i.e., excess Yang requiring dispersion. Drinking something will have the effect of lowering body temperature.

From his own experience the observant student will

know that when he feels cold, there are at least two ways of dealing with the situation. One can eat something, i.e., introduce Yang to balance the inner Yang deficiency — or one can empty the bladder, which disperses or drains off the excess Yin in the form of moisture.

Over and over again, especially when camping in winter conditions, we have noticed that a mouthful or two of food, even if the food is cold, has a more positive effect of restoring body temperature to normal than any amount of hot drinks.

Tension and Relaxation

ALL LIFE PROCESSES are to be considered as rhythmic or cyclic creations of polar tension and discharge of tension. There is always a continuous interplay of Yang and Yin — first one predominates, then the other. Stimulation is followed by discharge: activity is followed by repose: tension is followed by relaxation, just as night follows day and the seasons follow one another.

If the rhythmic period to a process is disturbed, then we have a condition requiring action to restore proper balance and rhythm. The rhythm may be too fast or too slow. There may be an excess of excitation which needs calming down or dispersing. The rhythm may be too slow, i.e., not enough stimulus, whether quantitive or qualitive, indicating a condition requiring stimulation, activation or, as the NEI CHING calls it, 'supplementing' action.

Let us consider a simple instance of a *local* symptom of excess Yang, and how, in accordance with FU HSI's formulation, appropriate treatment is to be applied. Consider a muscle in spasm. Prolonged firm pressure applied to an overtense muscle produces sudden relaxation of the muscle. This is a fact of observation familiar to physiotherapists.

We can understand why this happens if we apply

propositions 10 and 11.

A tense muscle is in a state of contraction, Yang. Pressure is a Yang stimulus. Like poles in close proximity repel one another. The stronger nullifies the weaker. There can be no discharge of tension between two polarities of like kind; thus for there to be a resolution ONE of these 'likes' must change. Either the therapists pressure must relax, become Yin, or the muscle resistance must relax, become Yin. The therapist maintains his pressure to the point where it produces a Yin re-action in the muscle. The muscle resistance (Yang) suddenly changes to the opposite pole, relaxation (Yin). The stronger annihilates the weaker. His pressure is now gently eased, being no longer needed. This example is also an instance of the application of the Hahnemannian principle of homoeopathy or treatment by a similar.

If the therapist uses an acupuncture needle locally, he would take 'draining' action, i.e., apply Yin to discharge the excess Yang.

ALL acupuncture treatment of symptoms, simple or complex syndromes and diseases, and ALL palliative treatments amount to re-equilibrizing polar process disturbances *already manifesting physically.* Assessment involves recognizing what particular process is disturbed: locating the site whereat it can be acted upon: and then acting upon it in the correct polarity. These then are three essentials: (a) Clear indication, (b) accurate location, (c) appropriate action.

Symptomatic treatment, or treatment of gross disturbances, belongs to the inferior doctor who has not enough knowledge or skill to prevent them from occurring. Symptom treatment does not eradicate root causes − it only palliates.

Five Elements Method

ALL illnesses, before they become outwardly, visibly or palpably manifested, have first an *invisible* stage, where Energy imbalances have not yet translated themselves from subtle levels into gross physical and physiological disturbances. The highest healing art and science deals with the invisible subtle level of energy disturbance, where illnesses and disease are only *potentially* physical. The traditional method for treating imbalances at this subtle level is known as the FIVE ELEMENTS METHOD. The family health practitioner should need no other method, except in rare emergencies.

When we talk of the FIVE ELEMENTS we do not mean 'elements' as material, but rather as conditions or stages. The ancient Greeks considered the primary conditions as four, namely, Earth, Air, Water, Fire. In India of the present day, as of old, only three 'elements' are taken as primary: Air, Fire, Water, or the Vayu, Pitta, and Kappa of the Tridosha system. Chinese tradition, in common with the Tibetan, consider five: Fire, Earth, Metal, Water, Wood.

We notice the omission of Air and the inclusion of two unfamiliar 'elements', Metal and Wood.

We do not need to feel disturbed or confused that some traditions include more 'elements' than do some others; or that they categorize them differently. We find differences in other classifications, as, for instance, the *Kingdoms of Nature.*

In the West, at the present day, there are only three Kingdoms of Nature ordinarily recognized as such: Mineral, Plant, Animal. According to others there are four or five Kingdoms. There appears to be a growing school of Western thought which considers there to be four distinct Kingdoms of nature: Mineral, Plant, Animal, Human.

The Tibetan Chi-Schara-Badgan doctrine inserts a class

between Plant and Animal, calling it the Sex-Differentiation Kingdom of Nature. The Tibetans also distinguish humans from animals, placing humans in the lowest rank of the CHI mode. Each classification has its own special merits. Our own personal preference leans towards the FIVE-divisioning, which seems to fit in best with the general medicine-philosophic ideas applicable to acupuncture. In an appendix we trace a brief outline, in the form of a 'family tree', of Creation from Nothing, through Analysis and Synthesis to FIVE Kingdoms of Nature. The table is by no means complete but is to be looked upon as suggestive and to stimulate further enquiry.

4.

Command Points

With each of the FIVE ELEMENTS of Chinese acupuncture there are associated certain inner organs, senses, sense-organs, tissues, systems, colours, flavours, emotions, heavenly bodies, cardinal points, seasons of the year, etc. All these associations indicate element-predominance-giving characteristic. Nothing is wholly any one element to the exclusion of the others. *Each has all five*, but one so predominates that it gives a one-element characteristic, and is named accordingly.

Thus, although we refer to the Stomach as an Earth organ, and the Kidneys as a Water organ, we must never lose sight of the fact that all inner organs are classified according to element dominance. All organs have traces of the four others, and it is through these traces that an organ is linked with other organs of a different element and with the main element's 'pool'. For example, the Metal organs, Lungs and Large Intestines, are linked through their Water element trace with the Water organs, Kidneys and Bladder: or through their Wood element trace with the Wood organs, Liver and Gall Bladder.

On each of the twelve superficial energy paths (the organ meridians) there is a special point which links the meridian's associated organ with one other organ. Each special point is named that other organ's element, e.g., the acupuncture point on the Heart meridian (a Fire organ) which links it with the Spleen (an Earth organ) is called the Earth point of the Heart meridian.

Each meridian has also a point on its path appropriate to its own organ's Element. The Elements and other special Command points are listed in full in the Table of Command Points. There is also a Table giving a short list of some of the principal five-divisioning correspondences.

TABLE I

THE COMMAND POINTS

Heart Meridian Meridian I	Small Intestine Meridian II	Circulation Meridian V	Three-Heater Meridian VI	Lung Meridian XI	Large Intestine Meridian X
Wood point .9	Metal point .1	Wood point .9	Metal point .1	Wood point .11	Metal point .1
Fire .8	Water .2	Fire .8	Water .2	Fire .10	Water .2
Earth & Source point .7	Wood .3	Earth & Source point .7	Wood .3	Earth & Source point .9	Wood .3
	Source .4		Source .4		Source .4
Passage point .5	Fire .5	Passage .6	Passage .5	Metal .7	Fire .5
Metal .4	Passage .7	Metal .5	Fire .6	Passage .7	Passage .6
Water .3	Earth .8	Water .3	Earth .10	Water .5	Earth .11

MERIDIANS OF THE ARM

(TABLE I (Continued)

Bladder meridian III	Kidneys meridian IV	Gall meridian VII	Liver meridian VIII	Stomach meridian XI	Spleen meridian XII
Earth .54	Water .10	Earth .34	Water .8	Earth .36	Water .9
Passage .58	Metal .7	Passage .37	Passage .5	Passage .40	Metal .5
Fire .60	Passage .4	Fire .38	Metal .4	Fire .41	Passage .4
Source .64	Earth & Source .3	Source .40	Earth & Source .3	Source .42	Earth & Source .3
Wood .65		Wood .41		Wood .43	
Water .66	Fire .2	Water .43	Fire .2	Water .44	Fire .2
Metal .67	Wood .1	Metal .44	Wood .1	Metal .45	Wood .1

MERIDIANS OF THE LEG

TABLE II

FIVE ELEMENTS CORRESPONDENCIES

Element	Wood	Fire	Earth	Metal	Water
Organs of Alimentation & Elimination	Gall VII	Small Intestine II	Stomach XI	Large Intestine X	Bladder III
Organs of Storage and Distribution	Liver VIII	Heart I	Spleen XII	Lungs IX	Kidneys IV
Colour	Green	Red	Yellow	White	Black
Season	Spring	Summer	Long Summer	Autumn	Winter
Direction in Space	East	South	Centre	West	North
Flavour	Sour	Bitter	Sweet	Hot Pungent Aromatic	Salty
Sense	Vision	Speech	Taste	Smell	Hearing
Sense Organ	Eyes	Mouth	Tongue	Nose	Ears
System or Tissues	Muscles Brain, Nerves	Vascular System	Flesh, Connective Tissue	Skin Hair	Bones
Emotion	Anger	Joy	Sympathy	Grief	Fear
Power	Birth & Growth	Maturity. Fulness	Decrease	Balance	Emptiness
Effect	gathering Astringent	Drying, Strengthening	Retarding	Dispersing Harmonizing	Softening
Characteristic Faculty, etc.	Spiritual Faculties	Divine Inspiration	Thoughts & Ideas	Lower Animal Spirits	Will & Resolution

Two Classes

Each Element has its own specially associated inner organ. (The organs, recognized as 'organs' by the ancients, are not all to which we are accustomed in Western medicine.) They are divided into two classes.

In the first we have the six organs whose function is that of Nutrition and Excretion (alimentation and elimination, the FU organs). These are concerned with the conversion of environmental matter into the individual's organic matter; and the throwing off of unassimilable matter and organic waste back into the environment.

These have been aptly called the 'Workshop' or 'Manufactory' organs, they are: Stomach, Large Intestine, Urinary Bladder, Gall Bladder, Small Intestine, and the Three-Heater organ. This last, the Three-Heater, is not recognized in Western medicine as an organ. This is the organ which according to the ancients, is concerned with the Temperature regulatory function, uniting into one the three systems which together are concerned with body temperature – the Uro-genital, Digestive, and Respiratory. In our view the traditional placing of the Three-Heater *sense* organ seems to equate it with that part of the Hypothalamus which rests upon the Circle of Willis, of the same tissue matrix as the optic nerves and retina, just posterior to the pituitary body. The Circle of Willis is so named after the English anatomist (1621-1675) and is the arterial circle, at the base of the brain, formed by the internal carotids and basilar arteries.*

In the next class of organs we have the six organs concerned with Energy Circulation, Storage, and Distribution (the TSANG organs). These are: Spleen, Lungs, Kidneys, Liver, Heart, Circulation. This last mentioned is again not looked upon as an organ in its own right in

* An article by us on this subject was published in *Fitness Magazine*, 1963.

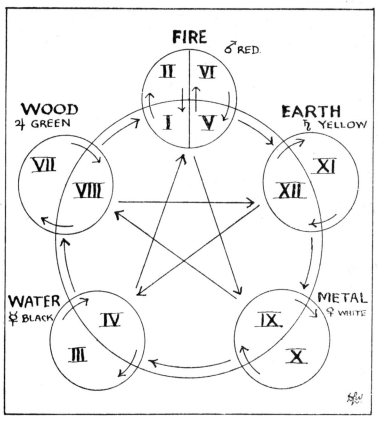

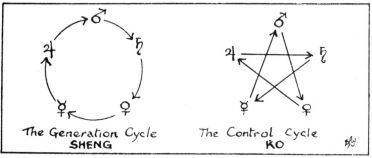

The Generation Cycle
SHENG

The Control Cycle
KO

Western medicine. The Circulation organ comprises the entire Vascular system. Some writers have called this organ the Vaso-Constrictor; others have named it the 'Heart surround'. This last name could be misleading for the Circulation organ of tradition is NOT the pericardium. Some authorities, especially those whose teachings are based upon Soulié de Morant, consider the Circulation organ to have special association with the Sex-function: other authorities consider the Sex-function as associated with the Water Element organ, the Kidneys.

To us the Sex-function seems more appropriately to be associated with the Kidneys, the general secernant organ of the whole body: in the sex act, one of excretion, the whole body passes in the seed.

5.

Five Element Cycles

THE FIVE ELEMENTS diagram represents the Elements, Earth, Metal, Water, Wood, Fire; the Organs associated with the Elements; the Colours said to belong to the Elements; and arrows indicating direction of flow of the Vital Energy.

There are two circuits shewn; these are the circuits which link the Storage and Distributory Organs with each other. One circuit links *adjacent* elements in what is known as the Generation Cycle (Sheng) or the Mother-Child.

Each Element is said to be the Child of the preceding and Mother of the succeeding Element, thus:

FIRE is the Mother of   EARTH and the Child of WOOD
EARTH is the Mother of METAL and the Child of FIRE
METAL is the Mother of WATER and the Child of EARTH
WATER is the Mother of WOOD and the Child of   METAL
WOOD is the Mother of   FIRE and the Child of   WATER

The generation cycle has easy-to-remember logical sequences, especially if one interprets the various Elements somewhat widely.

Fire produces ashes (earth); Earth (as ore) produces metal; Water produces Wood in the sense that water makes plant life possible; and Wood makes Fire in that Wood is fuel for Fire. The connection between Metal and Water is not so obvious. We get a line on the logic of this step through the Tibetan C-S-B, Metal is translated as AIR and as SLIME. Slime is a mixture of Earth and Water. If earth is separated out from the slime, water results. That is one way of considering things; another line of approach is the recognition that the MUCUS (slime) organs, Lungs and Large Intestine, are also AIR organs. The sense organ associated with the Element Metal is the Nose, with its sense of smell. Not only does mucous membrane come under the Metal Element but also the entire skin.

The other circuit, the Five-limbed STAR CYCLE is the cycle of 'Subjugates', 'Controls', 'Subdues' (KO). It is said that each Element in turn subjugates the next but one following, thus:

FIRE subjugates METAL (fire melts metal)
METAL subjugates WOOD (an axe fells a tree)
WOOD subjugates EARTH (primitive wooden implements till the soil)
EARTH subjugates WATER (earth absorbs water; earth dams or obstructs water flow)
WATER subjugates FIRE (water extinguishes fire).

There is another relationship known to tradition which we need to remember. This is called the relationship of 'endangers', or Husband-Wife, or Left hand-Right-hand relationship.

The Left side of the body is looked upon as the Yang side, or dominant side. In our diagram an organ shewn on the Left hand will, if deranged, *endanger* the organ on the Right hand shewn as linked by the arrow of the Control Cycle, thus:

The SMALL INTESTINE endangers the LARGE INTESTINE

The BLADDER endangers the THREE-HEATER
The GALL endangers the STOMACH
The HEART endangers the LUNGS
The LIVER endangers the SPLEEN
The KIDNEYS endanger the CIRCULATION.

If there is a derangement (of a left-hand organ) which continues for too long the right-hand organ WILL suffer. The natural consequence of disorder here causing disorder there is expressed, 'If the Husband is domineering and the wife is weak the result is tyranny; a weak husband and an extravagant wife leads to chaos.'

Though *both* classes of organ (Fu & Tsang) are influenced by the day and night rhythm and by the yearly seasons rhythm, the *intermittently functioning* organs of Nutrition and Excretion are more closely linked to the twenty-four hour cycle; and the *continuously functioning organs* of Distribution and Storage are more closely linked to the seasons.

Tidal Motion
Vital Energy has wave-like TIDAL motion; but not one tide only; several co-exist. In addition to the two just mentioned, the daily and the yearly, there is yet a third energy tide coinciding with lunations, or 'influence of the moon'.

One of the effects of the Tides is that there are best times for influencing the Energy; and therefore, according to the goal desired so the practitioner chooses an appropriate period of increase or decrease, maximum or minimum activity, in other words, he treats at the right time. Certain precautions and prohibitions regarding treatment are linked with these various Tides, as for example, Do not drain when the moon is empty: Supplement in the morning when Yang is on the increase, etc.

This notion of waves and tides is important, for it emphasizes something we indicated earlier: Energy equilibra are not static or unchanging states. Properly balanced energies means that changes are happening at a proper rate.

If a process is going on at the speed it should, then the balance is a dynamic one. If a change is too fast or too slow it is out of balance. An unbalance means there is either EXCESS or DEFICIENCY. The Five Elements method then is a method of equilibrizing element energies.

Transfer of Energy

The principle that *must* be observed is that in order to effect a balance, *Energy is to be transferred from where there is too much to where there is too little.*

One does certainly not set about getting rid of Excess through dispersing it into thin air, and then trying to supply a deficiency from some outside source.

Clearly the most economical way is to effect a transfer from where there is more to where there is less. So we come to an important rule: Always act upon the Deficiency by drawing upon the Excess. 'Waste not, want not' is a maxim that applies to Vital Energy resources as thoroughly as it can apply anywhere else! Longevity itself depends upon observance of this rule.

The expressions 'Excess' and 'Deficiency' can best be looked upon as equivalent to Hyper- and Hypo-activity, rather than to an organ being full or empty of material.

A large intestine showing Deficiency (by Pulse diagnosis) means that it is deficient in activity and thus might well be congested or full of excrementitious matter. Symptoms indicative of EXCESS include Pain, Heat, Spasm, over-activity; whereas symptoms of DEFICIENCY include Asthenia, Cold, Paralysis, underactivity, etc.

There is a ONE WAY ONLY flow through the meridians and through the inter-organ channels. This direction is indicated schematically by the arrows in our Five Elements diagram. Life Energy MUST travel in the direction shewn. Flow in the opposite direction spells DEATH. Nourishment must flow from mother to child, not in the reverse direction.

Spleen Deficiency
For example if a Deficiency shows on the Spleen and an Excess on the Heart this means that in order to bring about a re-balance the Excess must be drawn along its natural path in the direction of the arrow, in this case the Mother to Child path. This is done by taking SUPPLY action at the FIRE POINT of the Spleen.

If, however, the Deficiency on the Spleen occurs with the Excess on the Lungs the rebalancing path will NOT be the Mother-Child path between Spleen and Lung. Excess cannot flow from Metal to Earth in the direction opposite to the natural generation flow. This becomes obvious when we say, as with the Chinese, 'If the child is hungry give it the breast — but if the mother is hungry you do not give her the child to eat'. In this case the Excess will need to be drawn along natural paths, in the direction of the arrows, by the most economical route, namely to the Spleen from WOOD, and to WOOD from Metal. It could, of course travel the longer way round, all round the generation cycle. Any combination of Generation and Control cycles may be used. The only essential condition is that Energy must be drawn in the direction of flow to SUPPLY the Deficiency. As an item of 'Artistry' in treatment the general guiding principle of economy is followed, 'Never use more needles than are necessary'. In the case above, action is first taken on the WOOD point of the Spleen meridian, then on the METAL point of the Liver meridian. As the student will see we have first SUPPLEMENTED at the Deficiency (on the Spleen) drawing upon a NORMAL organ – this action *creates* a small deficiency on the Wood organ, the Liver, upon which we can now take supply action to draw off the Excess from the lungs. This we do at the Metal point of the Liver.

In this example just given, we were concerned with two YIN or Storage organs which are directly linked along the Generation and the Control Cycle pathways. The Yang organs are not directly linked in the same way along the Generation and Control paths; the links have to be made through the intermediary of special channels which link the organs of a pair. Note that each YIN organ meridian is paired with a YANG organ meridian.

Act Upon the Deficiency

Suppose we have a Deficiency on the Stomach (Earth) and Excess on the Small Intestine (Fire). Applying always the rule 'Act upon the Deficiency', the connecting channel which links the Stomach and Spleen meridians is opened or activated so that Energy is drawn into the Stomach from the Spleen. The acupuncture point used to effect this is known as *The Passage point on the Stomach meridian.* This action induces a small deficiency on the Spleen, upon which we can now act at the Fire point to draw Energy from the Fire organs. The deficiency now induced on the Heart meridian is acted upon by taking Supply action on the Passage point of the Heart. This opens the channel enabling the Excess from the Small Intestine to flow through the natural paths (now freed or stimulated) to the Stomach.

Diagrammatically speaking, Energy is drawn across the circle barrier, inwards or outwards, through Passage points.

Each of the twelve organ meridians has on its path an acupuncture point said to have direct linkage with the meridian *organ*, or source of that meridian's energy. Hence this point is called the *Source Point*, it is also known (according to different authors and/or schools) as the *Organ point, Prime Mover, Regulator Point*, etc. *ON all the YIN meridians this point co-incides with the EARTH Point.* On the Yang meridians the Source or Organ Point is a separate point.

The Source (organ) points are acted upon if the meridian's associated organ itself is affected. These points may be used by themselves or in conjunction with other Elements points, in order to re-inforce their action. This is why they are sometimes known as the Re-inforcement points.

Deficiencies without Excess

So far we have only dealt with instances of restoration of Normal balance by transfer or 're-shuffle'. This should always be our aim; re-balance by transfer. Nevertheless cases occur where a Deficiency shows up, but NO Excess anywhere upon which to draw; or an Excess may show without there being any Deficiency into which it may be drained.

When we come across Deficiencies and NO Excess upon which to draw, then Energy needs to be brought in from outside. This condition is very common at the present day, and, in our view, is largely caused by the poor quality food consumed. In general a careful attention to diet will bring Vitality up to what it should be. Foods are to be selected appropriate to the Element showing Deficiency. This is a use of the FIVE FLAVOURS.

If there are Excesses without Deficiences into which they may be drained, we still have to apply the rule Waste not want not. We do not therefore drain off the surplus and dispel it into thin air. We induce a small deficiency, or allow a small deficiency to build, this will usually be done in the Generation Cycle on the 'child' of the Excess. The inducing of a deficiency is not done by needles, nor for that matter, by any action at acupuncture points. Quite simple means are used, namely: A short fast creates a deficiency on the Stomach: a long fast creates a deficiency on the Small intestine: urination creates a small deficiency on the Bladder, etc. Thus we have therapeutic application of dieting, sweating, aperients, reduction of fats in the diet, and general diet regulation, etc.

6.

Meridians

RE-BALANCING OF THE VITAL ENERGY as it circulates in the Inner organs is effected by acupuncture
treatment at certain surface points on the peripheral
circuits known as the Meridians. There are twelve of these.
The Twelve organ Meridians follow well-established and
clearly defined paths. The circulation of Energy is *continuous*, and thus one cannot say that the circulation
begins anywhere; it is only for convenience of description
that we begin our description of the surface paths with the
first point on the Heart Meridian. In this we follow the
numbering of meridians now generally accepted in Western
culture.

Some authors begin their numbering with the Lungs
meridian, but, as we see it, there is no valid reason for
asserting that this is more logical. From some points of
view the Heart appears more logical in that the heart beats
many months before the lungs come into action.

In ANY circular process it is a matter of preference
where one arbitrarily elects to 'begin'. It is necessary only
to consider any analogous example, such as the continuous
transition from Day to Night and Night to Day. When does
one day end, and the new day begin? Noon? Midnight?
Dawn? Sunset?

Practically all European schools of acupuncture of any
significance begin their numbering of the meridians with

the Heart as 1. In this book, as in our first, we use Roman numerals to indicate Meridians and arabic numbers to indicate the acupuncture point numbers. It is easier to become accustomed to remembering the meridians by a Roman number than by naming it in full (or using letter symbols). For optimum efficiency of international communication, standardization is important. We stressed this in our earlier work, pointing out the confusion of symbolism already existing in 1959.

I. THE HEART MERIDIAN. This meridian begins on the thorax, right up in the apex of the axilla. Even more exactly described, the first point is below the outer border of the first rib, on the axillary artery where this can be felt pulsating between the subscapularis and the coraco-brachialis muscles, and the tendons of the latissimus dorsi. The path of the meridian goes down the arm and forearm antero-medially to finish at the root of the little finger nail. There are in all NINE acupuncture points on this meridian.

II. *THE SMALL INTESTINE MERIDIAN.* This has its first point on the little finger at the root of the finger nail, the path travels up the postero-internal aspect of the arm, over the shoulder to the face where it has its nineteenth and last point just anterior to the tragus. There are in all NINETEEN acupuncture points on this meridian.

III. *THE BLADDER MERIDIAN.* This meridian has its first point on the face, just medial to the inner corner of the eye. From the eye the path goes over the top of the head to the back of the neck, down the back, and the back of the thighs, legs, and outer border of the foot to finish at the root of the little toe nail. There are in all SIXTY-SEVEN acupuncture points on the Bladder meridian.

IV. *THE KIDNEYS MERIDIAN.* This meridian begins on the sole of the foot, the first point between the two large pads formed at the base of the big toe and other toes. The path then travels up the internal aspect of leg and thigh to the groin, up the anterior of the abdomen and thorax to finish just below the clavicle in the triangular hollow formed by the first rib, clavicle, and sternum. There are in all TWENTY-SEVEN acupuncture points on the Kidneys meridian.

V. *THE CIRCULATION MERIDIAN.* The meridian begins on the thorax, just lateral to the nipple, goes to the arm, down the anterior of arm and forearm, over the palm of the hand to finish at the root of the nail of the middle finger. It is to be noted that this is the only meridian which has no forbidden points. There are in all NINE acupuncture points on the Circulation meridian.

VI. *THE THREE-HEATER MERIDIAN.* This meridian, which is sometimes called the THERMO-REGULATOR, begins with its first point at the root of the nail of the ring finger, the path goes over the back of the hand, up the forearm, arm, over the back of the shoulder to the side of the neck, round the ear to the 23rd and last point just close to the outer extremity of the eyebrow. There are in all TWENTY-THREE acupuncture points on the Three-Heater meridian.

VII. *THE GALL BLADDER or GALL MERIDIAN.* This meridian starts with its first point just behind the outer corner of the eye, vertically below the last point of the Three-Heater meridian. The path goes back and forth over the skull and back to the nape of the neck, forward over the shoulder, down the side of the thorax and abdomen, outer side of the thigh and leg to finish at the root of the fourth toe-nail. There are in all FORTY-FOUR acupuncture points on the Gall meridian.

VIII. *THE LIVER MERIDIAN.* The Liver meridian begins near the root of the big toe-nail (2nd toe side), the path goes up the inner aspect of the leg and thigh, over the abdomen to finish on the costal border (where this is intersected by a vertical line drawn down from the nipple). On this meridian there are in all FOURTEEN acupuncture points.

IX. *THE LUNGS MERIDIAN*. This meridian begins with its first point in the first intercostal space on the continuation of the paraxillary line. The path goes down the antero-lateral aspect of the arm to the last point at the root of the thumb nail. There are in all ELEVEN acupuncture points on the Lungs meridian. . . . . ,

X. *THE LARGE INTESTINE* or *COLON MERIDIAN*. This meridian pathway has its first point at the root of the nail of the index finger, the path travels up the postero-lateral of the forearm and arm, over the shoulder, neck and face to the last point at the side of the nostril. There are in all TWENTY acupuncture points on this meridian.

XI. *THE STOMACH MERIDIAN*. Most European authorities consider the Stomach meridian as beginning on the forehead, at what Dr Wu Wei Ping calls the 8th point. He treats this meridian as having the first point on the face at the centre of the lower edge of the orbital cavity, vertically below the centre of the pupil. From the face the path travels down the throat to the front of the thorax and abdomen to the anterior of the thigh and leg to finish at the root of the nail of the second toe. There are in all FORTY-FIVE acupuncture points on this meridian.

XII. *THE SPLEEN MERIDIAN*. This begins at the root of the big toe-nail (medial side) the path goes up the internal aspect of leg and thigh, crosses the groin up the abdomen and thorax to finish in the sixth intercostal space in the axillary line. There are in all TWENTY-ONE acupuncture points on the Spleen meridian.

Vessel Meridians
In addition to the twelve organ meridians there are two Vessel meridians that are often classified as meridians XIII

and XIV. We do not indicate these two Vessel meridians
by a number but by their names in full. They are
sufficiently different from the Organ meridians that they
should not be confused with them as forming part of the
organ meridian system; yet they have certain characteristics closely allied to the organ Meridians. These two
Vessel meridians are known as the CONCEPTION and the
GOVERNOR Vessels. The Conception Vessel has its first
point in the exact centre of the perineum. The path
follows the anterior median line up the abdomen, thorax,
throat to just below the lower lip. There are in all
TWENTY-FOUR acupuncture points on the Conception
meridian. The Governor Vessel has its first point at the tip
of the coccyx, the path follows the posterior median line
the full length of the spine, over the skull, to finish inside
the mouth on the front of the upper gum between the
roots of the two front teeth.

The Circuit in the Organ meridian system exhibits
certain polar changes, thus: the Energy travelling from the
thorax to finger tip is YIN predominant energy, as the
energy approaches the extremity the polarity begins to
change, and by the time the tip of the finger is reached
YIN dominance is extinguished and YANG dominance
begins. Energy travelling from finger-tips to the face and
from the face to the toes is characterized as YANG
dominant energy. As the Energy approaches the lower
extremity the polarity begins to change. By the time the
extremities of the toes are reached YANG dominance has
become extinguished and on the journey from the toes to
the thorax the YIN becomes dominant.

Note that it is at the extremities of the upper and lower
limbs that the vital energy changes polarity. In the central
area, head and thorax, even though the energy passes from
one meridian to another, there is no polarity change.

The polarity change is not sudden, but occurs between

the elbow and finger tips, and between the knee and toes. *It is at points below the knee and below the elbow that polarity change can be most easily retarded or accelerated* — it is therefore within these limits that the most important CONTROL or COMMAND POINTS will be found. In our charts, where the five elements points are marked, they will be found at or below the knee, at or below the elbow. As a form of 'shorthand' on the charts, we have used certain conventional signs as used in astronomy to indicate heavenly bodies. The Five Elements have each an associated heavenly body, thus:

WOOD	FIRE	EARTH	METAL	WATER
Jupiter	Mars	Saturn	Venus	Mercury
♃	♂	♄	♀	☿

Footnote:

It would be well for the student to become accustomed to making his notes (case sheets, etc.,) using a standard form of shorthand or symbols. We have found the following symbols to serve very well, they are easy to write and to recognize.

I–XII, roman numerals to indicate MERIDIAN

.1–.67,   a point followed by arabic number to indicate the acupuncture point number.

If the acupuncture point is a Command Point this is then indicated by the use of the following symbols.

♃ = Wood point   ♀ = Metal point   LO = passage point

♂ = Fire point   ☿ = Water point

♄ = Earth point   ° = Organ point

These signs are then followed, if necessary by a symbol indicating where the point is forbidden to needle or to moxa, thus:

▢ = forbidden to needle   △ = forbidden to moxa.

Examples:

II·34 =   The small intestine meridian third point is the Wood point of that meridian.

VI·5 LO =   Three-heater meridian point number five is the Passage (Lo point) point of that meridian.

$\text{IX} \cdot 8^{?\Delta}_{\dagger} =$ Lungs meridian, point eight, Metal point, forbidden to Moxa.

$\text{XII} \cdot 3^{\circ}_{b} =$ Spleen meridian third point is the Earth point and Organ (Source) point.

We now come to the question: How does the practitioner assess the state of balance of the Five Elements — or the state of organ function associated with each element, etc.

There are many ways. This is especially so when an Excess or Deficiency has persisted for long enough to externalize in outwardly detectable symptoms. In these cases the COLOUR of the skin, excretions, exudats, secretions, and so on will indicate excess or deficiency of the associated Element.

The PSYCHOLOGICAL state will also be found of inestimable value, especially in the detection of imbalances in the very early stages, before the symptoms develop outwardly. We have personally found the psychological state to be a more subtle, readable and reliable guide than the pulses. The pulses are generally looked upon as constituting the characteristic diagnostic technique. (The psychological considerations are dealt with later).

7.

Pulses

Thousands of years before the Christian era the Chinese recognized that there was a definite relationship between the heart-beat, respiration rate and blood flow. This relationship reflected the state of health of the *organism as a whole.* This is acknowledged in Western medicine, and it is an essential part of clinical examination to note breathing rate, whether deep or shallow, even or irregular, easy, laboured, etc. How many heart-beats to the breath, etc.

To most Westerners, when one mentions, 'Taking a patient's pulse', attention goes at once to the wrist where the radial artery is easily felt pulsating. There are several other places where the pulsations could as easily be felt; in fact wherever an artery runs close to a bone and close to the surface.

Diagnosis through the Pulses
The truly great discovery made (as far as we know) by the Chinese was that *through the pulses it is possible to read not merely the health of the organism as a whole but also that of each inner organ separately.* Whether it has much or little energy; whether congested, overfull, or escaping, deficient; whether hyper- or hypo-active; whether the polarity' predominance and the polar changes are what they should be, etc. The Chinese discovered, quite early in

their medicine-history, that at the wrist there were twelve distinctly discernible pulses. That is to say upon each wrist there were three positions, and at each position two levels. A different inner state reflected at each of the pulses.

If the reader intends ever to practise acupuncture, when pulses will be significant, he will have to feel inwardly deeply convinced that pulses technique makes sense, and that two levels at three positions can give distinctive and different readings. He will have to test and experience the fact of difference for himself.

A simple laboratory experiment can be made to illustrate the reality of differences. If we have a fluid flowing through a resilient tube (rubber or plastic attached to a water tap) and we *very lightly touch* the tube with a finger the flow can be felt. That is to say one can feel quite definitely the fact of flow when there is the merest delicate touch. Let the fingertip linger a while so that the *kind of sensation* registers: now steadily compress the tube, increasing the pressure until the flow has become almost stopped, then lift ever so slightly and continue to feel at this level. You will notice that the kind of sensation now in the finger tip is different from that of the first light touch.

The experiment is continued by varying the surface upon which the tube rests. A tube resting upon a hard surface will feel different from when it is resting upon a soft surface. There will also be a difference if one places a layer of material between finger and tube. If you do try this out you will soon recognize that it is far from nonsensical to suggest that a pulse felt superficially in one place can give a noticeably different reading from a pulse position only a fingerswidth away.

Our chart illustrates the traditional pulses positions and organs to which they correspond.

Assessing One's Own Pulses

The student begins by learning to read and assess his own pulses, for, according to tradition, the pulses of the practitioner are taken as his standard, and therefore a practitioner MUST HIMSELF BE IN GOOD HEALTH. The healer sets an example to the patient. It is an accepted rule that a practitioner in poor health does not give acupuncture treatment: in any case how could he diagnose?

In order to take his own pulse the practitioner sits relaxed. To read the pulses of his *left* hand he rests the back of his left wrist on the palm of the right hand and curls the fingers over so that the tops rest on the radial artery. The middle finger is placed at the level of the bony prominence just below the wrist fold. This is called the BAR pulse position. 'Bar' names the bony prominence and does not in any way imply a barrier as some translators seem to infer. The forefinger will then rest naturally on the fold itself at the base of the thenar eminence. This position is called the INCH or POUCE position. 'Inch' is but another translation to mean *Thenar* or *Thumb* position. The ring finger again will fall naturally into the correct third position known as the CUBIT.

On the Left Hand

POSITION 1: the 'Inch' is the position nearest to the thumb, and is felt with the forefinger.

POSITION 2: the 'Bar' is felt with the middle finger.

POSITION 3: the 'Cubit' is felt with the ring finger.

Light pressure at position 1 detects the superficial pulse which is the Pulse of the SMALL INTESTINE. *Deep* pressure reveals the deep pulse, which is that of the HEART.

Light pressure at position 2 detects the superficial pulse,

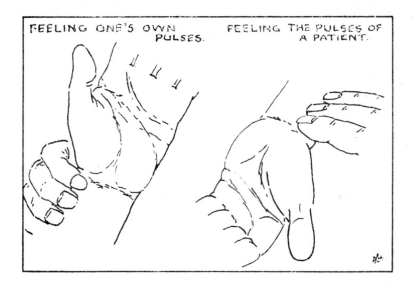

FEELING ONE'S OWN PULSES.   FEELING THE PULSES OF A PATIENT.

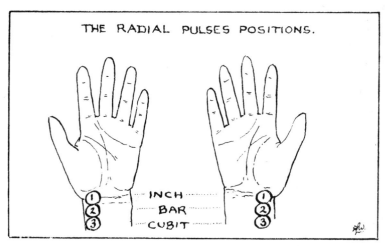

THE RADIAL PULSES POSITIONS.

① ② ③   INCH ...... BAR ...... CUBIT ......   ① ② ③

which is the pulse of the GALL BLADDER; while *deep* pressure here reveals the deep pulse which is that of the LIVER.

Light pressure at position 3 detects the superficial pulse which is the pulse of the BLADDER; *deep* pressure here reveals the deep pulse, which is that of the KIDNEYS.

The superficial pulses are those of the YANG, while the deep pulses are those of the YIN.

The same method will apply when taking the pulses *on the Right Hand.*

POSITION 1: the 'Inch' Superficial LARGE INTEST-INE Deep LUNGS.

POSITION 2: the 'Bar' Superficial STOMACH Deep SPLEEN.

POSITION 3: the 'Cubit' Superficial THREE-HEATER Deep CIRCULATION.

All superficial pulses relate to YANG, deep to YIN ORGANS.

In general it may safely be said that only a very little practice suffices to detect differences; but it takes a long time and a great deal of practice to become proficient in reading and interpreting the pulses with any high degree of skill and artistry.

If one or more of the pulses is scarcely discernible, this does not necessarily indicate a disturbance – on the contrary it may indicate that that particular pulse, at that hour of the day, at that season of the year, and in relation to other circumstances, is as it should be.

The Chinese allotted a number, a sort of score, to each of the pulse readings. 4 is taken as the normal. On the YIN or deficient side the score ranges 3-2-1-0 (with a score of 0 the patient is as good as dead). A score of 3 indicates deficiency sufficient to warrant action, though there might not necessarily be any other symptom than that of the pulse itself. On the Yang side the score ranges 5-6-7-8. Here the score of 8 would again represent a patient *in extremis.*

When feeling the pulses the practitioner 'listens' to them much as one listens to an orchestra — each pulse representing one of the instrumentalists. Taken all together the 'melody' should be a happy and harmonious one. It is as if one is listening to that person's 'life-song'. If the melody is not joyous and harmonious at least one of the players is out of tune. The practitioner needs to locate which is the discordant player.

Pulses assessment is not a matter to be approached roughly and without sensitivity. A highly important rule to be observed is SILENCE WHILE READING THE PULSES.

Assessing Patient's Pulses

To read the patient's pulses, the practitioner rests the patient's left hand in his left hand and palpates with his right, and vice versa for the right hand pulses. The patient should be relaxed and have rested for *at least ten minutes,* preferably longer, to allow time for the calming down of any emotional excitement or physical exertion which would otherwise tend to give misleading readings.

The Chinese considered the ideal time for taking the pulses readings as between 5 a.m. and 1 p.m. But for obvious reasons this is not always workable, especially with a busy practice. Various factors have to be taken into account when reading the pulses; the time of day is one of them.

The patient should be comfortably reclining and NOT hopping from one foot to the other. A master *might* be able to arrive at a pulses assessment within a few minutes, the patient standing and chatting away — but more often than not if you ever see a pulse being taken in this way, you may safely assume the practitioner is no master, and whatever readings he gets would represent a highly unreliable set of information items.

The practitioner himself must be relaxed, calm and receptive. When he palpates at each position, at each level, he quite deliberately silently says to himself, for example, 'I am now listening to the pulse of the Small Intestine to hear and try to understand what it is saying to me'.

This almost ritual approach to the pulses has often been sneered at by Westerners who understand so little of Far-Eastern wisdom. It does not matter if it takes a whole hour to assess the pulses. It does not matter if, in that hour, the pulses are read and re-read several times. It is important to cultivate the ability to listen to the vital message which will become clearly revealed to the calm and *receptive* mind. If this hour is followed by thirty seconds of treatment at the right place, more good will be done for the patient than if thirty seconds of diagnosis is followed by an hour of treatment.

What is the Life Force doing in each one of the Organs and Organ Meridians? Is there so little vital energy that it speaks in the pulse as if it were a thin drawn silk thread? Is the energy hurriedly pouring itself away and, as it were, 'the sands rapidly running out'? Is there somewhere a blockage against which the Life Force is striving to push its way? Is the life-effort erratic?

The Pulses Cannot Lie
The human being *will*, through the pulses, tell the inmost secrets of the Life Force animating it, and its message will be a truthful message. If the practitioner is sincere and genuinely seeks to understand and receive the message, it will be there. Life always speaks truth about itself — one simply needs to learn at what level to listen. The practitioner, then, listens with open mind and eager

sympathetic heart. He accepts what he reads, for his task is to read the message as the Life Force in the patient gives it.

The pulses indicate not only whether an organ is hyper- or hypo-active, has excess or deficiency of energy, they also indicate whether an organ is physiologically full or empty. This may readily be tested. Read the Bladder pulse before and after urination; read the Large Intestine pulse before and after an evacuation; read the Stomach pulse before and after a meal.

One practitioner of our acquaintance told us, with a certain amount of self-satisfaction over his prowess at reading the Chinese Pulses, 'I can always find a deficiency on the Bladder Meridian, so I make it a rule to tone up the bladder at the first treatment,' Of course he always found that, for the simple reason there was a toilet between the dressing-room and consulting room, patients seldom omitted to call in on the way.

8.

Treatment Techniques

TREATMENT TECHNIQUES: The term 'acupuncture' which literally means 'pricking with a needle' tends to be misleading. It gives the impression that the needle technique is the one and only. There are several ways of bringing about the desired effect: the three principal ways are MASSAGE, MOXA, and NEEDLE. All three are equally effective.

We have so far not come across any explanation of the therapeutic techniques as regards their manner of functioning that is to us completely satisfying. It is difficult to be able to say with scientific precision just what state, condition or phenomenon it is that we are dealing with in acupuncture. Until some big advance is made and a theory put forward that will be capable of explaining apparent contradictions and problems, the most satisfactory basis upon which we can think and work is that *Vital Energy represents some form of Electricity.*

This does not mean that vital energy *is* electricity, but that its behaviour, responses, reactions, etc., are such as to indicate that many of the laws applying to electricity also apply to Vital Energy.

It also appears to us, as we wrote in an appendix to our earlier work, that vital energy manifestations are closely linked with colloids and colloidal behaviour. Our notes on this were first published in 1959; in the ensuing years we have devoted much reflective thought to this problem, and to-day (1965) still feel that it is in the 'collodial' direction that we should look for a workable theory.

Colloidal Behaviour

In order that the reader may understand this basis we go briefly into the subject of colloids and colloidal behaviour, in simple non-technical terms. This does not by any means imply wandering away from the subject, acupuncture, but on the contrary we shall simply be making deeper enquiry into the HOW of acupuncture than is customary among teachers of acupuncture. In our view it is not enough for a practitioner to 'go through the motions' of a treatment technique: for unless there is sufficient understanding of what is happening he will, sooner or later be faced with a treatment problem to which *no answer is to be found in any text book,* and *only his own understanding will enable him to work out a solution.*

Between the smallest visible particle and the molecular size is the size range sometimes referred to as the 'twilight zone of matter'. It is within this range that 'colloidal behaviour' happens. A colloid occurs when very fine particles of one material are suspended in other media, which may be gaseous or liquid, the particles themselves may be gaseous, liquid or solid.

A simple form of colloid can be exemplified in an *emulsion* where we have droplets of, let us say, some oily matter suspended in a watery medium. With some emulsions the minute oily droplets will remain in suspension more or less indefinitely; with other emulsions the tendency for the droplets to coalesce and settle is such that the emulsion is highly unstable. *Emulsions* are colloids occurring as particles of solids or liquids in liquid media. There are also colloids as particles of solid matter in gaseous media, *Smokes;* and liquids in gaseous media, *Mists.*

Two Phases

In every colloid there are two tendencies or phases. There is the tendency for the finely divided particles to *repel* one another (remain apart), and there is the tendency for the particles to coalesce or join up with neighbouring particles. These two phases are known in colloidal chemistry as the SOL and GEL phases. The SOL phase labels the tendency to stay finely divided, or to increase subdivision; the GEL phase labels the tendency to unite into larger units eventually causing cessation of the 'colloid' state. A colloid is said to be DEAD when SOL has become *irreversibly* GEL.

All colloids are unstable, but some far more so than others. As the state moves towards increase GEL the colloid is said to *age*. In some colloids the ageing process is reversible, and the changes take the form of changes in viscosity. Some changes are slow, some are rapid.

It is scientifically accepted that *ALL LIFE HAPPENS only where there is PROTOPLASM BEHAVING COLLOIDALLY.*

In living structures the colloids are extremely sensitive with enormous possibilities as regards potential stability, reversibility of phase, etc. One of the characteristics of Life is periodicity or rhythmicity; in other words fluctuation between predominencies of SOL and GEL phases. All colloids, very much so living colloids, are electrically sensitive. Alfred Korzybski calls colloidal behaviour a physico-electro-chemical occurrence. Living systems depend for their rhythmic behaviour upon the chemically alterable film (surface tension film behaving as a membrane) which divides the electrically conducting phases. Living organisms can be described as film-bounded and partitioned irritable systems: which is to say 'sensitive to electrical currents'.

Disturbance of Colloidal Balance

There are several factors which can disturb or change colloidal balance (structure), that is to say, accelerate or retard one phase or another: for example *all known forms of radiant energy* can effect colloids.

In an organism living in health, the complex totality of manifold colloidal structures behave with *appropriate periodicity* and rhythm between certain phase limits. Any phase of any of the colloidal systems which goes beyond the appropriate limit, or fails to reach the limit within the proper time, *will affect the health of the organism-as-a-whole. Likewise any* factor, intrinsic or extrinsic, capable of altering colloidal behaviour *will have a marked effect* one way or another upon the welfare of the organism.

Korzybski has pointed out that the action of all drugs is based upon their effect on colloidal equilibrium: it is well known that various acids or alkalis change the electrical resistance of protoplasm. He has also stressed this very important point (important to us in acupuncture) that *physical* colloidal states go paired with nervous, mental, and other characteristics, and that *all illnesses are somehow connected with colloidal disturbances.* He writes:

'By structural necessity, every expression of cellular activity involves some sort of colloidal behaviour; and any factor disturbing the colloidal structure must be disturbing to the welfare of the organism. Vice versa, a factor which is beneficial to the organism must reach and affect the colloids.'

(Note carefully these last fourteen words.)

Summation of Colloidal Behaviour

We sum up in four sentences:

Colloidal behaviour is exhibited by materials of a very fine sub-division which involves *surface activities and electrical characteristics.*

All life processes involve *at least* electrical currents.

Electrical currents *and other forms of energy* are able to affect the colloidal structures upon which our physical characteristics depend, i.e., they influence our bodies and our minds.

All life is characterized by protoplasm behaving colloidally.

From the above it will be clearly seen that, as regards acupuncture treatment techniques, *whether one uses massage, moxa, or needles therapeutic use is being made of one of the factors able to alter collodial equilibrium.* This will become even more obvious if we list these various factors in a way similar to that done by Korzybski. There are four main factors, followed by a fifth which Korzybski shewed to apply *only to human beings.*

1. PHYSICAL e.g., x-rays, radium, ultra-violet rays, light, heat, electricity, cathode rays, and in fact *all* radiant energy.
2. MECHANICAL e.g., friction, puncture, pressure, percussion, sound and ultra-son.
3. BIOLOGICAL e.g., microbes, parasites, sperm, etc.
4. CHEMICAL e.g., drugs, poisons, and *some* foods.

The fifth factor which applies only to human beings has been labelled by Korzybski 'semantic re-actions' meaning re-action to symbols in connection with their meaning; we therefore call this factor *2-em.*

5. SYMBOLIC or PSYCHIC. What is going on in the patient's mind influences his own colloidal state. What is going on in the practitioner's mind is also therapeutically significant. In other words the practitioner's INTENTION has great influence upon the quality and polarity treatment he will in fact administer.*

* For further study of colloids see Chapter IX of Alfred Korzybski's *Science and Sanity*, and Dr Majorie Swanson's monograph *Scientific and Epistemologic Backgrounds of General Semantics*, both published by G. S. Institute, Lakeville, Conn, U.S.A.

9.

Massage

Though there are several massage techniques there are only two polarities of treatment. The different techniques all have this in common, namely, ability to accelerate, retard, or even reverse SOL/GEL phases. We refer to the treatment polarities as YIN or YANG as explained below.

EXCESS energy, hypertonicity, hyperactivity, hyper-secretion, pain, spasm, etc., require YIN action, or draining, dispersion, sedation, soothing, relaxing, calming, or other suitable synonym. In the NEI CHING the expression used for this polarity action is DRAINING.

DEFICIENCY of energy, hypotonicity, hypo-activity, hypo-secretion, torpid, sluggish, paralytic states require YANG action, or toning, stimulating, supplying, activating, focusing, enlivening, vitalizing, etc. The NEI CHING refers to this polarity action as SUPPLEMENTING.

Massage techniques for supplementing and draining include the following:

(i) Use of a special massage instrument or 'needle',

(ii) Use of finger-nail for friction or pressure,

(iii) Use of fingers for friction, pressure, movement,

(iv) Use of knuckles and elbows for pressure and movement,

(v) Use of knuckles, elbows, toes, knees, and the heel of the hand for percussion.

Massage Needles

The traditional massage instrument is in the form of an ivory or bone needle, ending not in a point but in a ball. The essential characteristic of the instrument is that part which comes into contact with the patient's flesh shall be of an electrically insulating, non-conducting material such as ivory, bone, ebony, bakelite, plastic, etc.

A light, rapid, uni-directional friction upon a dry surface with such an instrument causes a small static charge to build up which, on attaining a certain magnitude, will discharge itself. It has been demonstrated with various electrical instruments that acupuncture points coincide with small areas of low electrical resistance (high conductivity) relative to the lower conductivity of the surrounding tissues.

A charge built up in the vicinity of an acupuncture point will, upon discharging itself, be released at the point of lowest electrical resistance. The static charge is extremely small, but it is its very minuteness that gives it penetration power to reach the inner organs or relevant colloidal structure. This light, rapid, unidirectional movement represents the YANG polarity treatment to tone, stimulate, activate, supplement, etc.

Using the same instrument the opposite polarity of treatment to drain or disperse an accumulated charge or excess, is by relatively slow, steady, firm movements of a 'spreading' nature.

Alternatives to Needles

The Chinese practitioner would often use his finger-nail in lieu of the bone needle, for the nail, being of a bony or horny substance, is electrically insulating. Provided that the finger-nails are long enough to ensure that only the nail comes into contact with the patient's skin, this serves as an effective instrument.

Pressure, whether with the finger-nail, finger-tip, or other part, is applied in two polarities. Where there is an excess to be drained or dispersed, pressure is applied gradually, firmly, increasing until heavy pressure is reached, which is maintained until the operator *feels* a relaxation in the tissues. Pressure is then released very slowly, indeed almost imperceptibly.

The supplementing movement pressure is applied rapidly to the desired depth and, as soon as the tissues respond, (which will be felt as an increase in tension) pressure is quickly removed. Several applications may be needed before the tissues respond, thus we could describe this action as a 'pumping' action.

When the fingers are moved in deep friction and kneading it is our personal opinion that the 'Fifth factor' plays considerable part, for the following reasons. It is already scientifically established that a muscle in action emits radio waves. The radio waves are *stronger* from the *smaller* muscles; this applies especially to the small muscles of the fingers and hand, e.g., the lumbricales. In our view the quality and intensity of the radiations from the operator's muscles are directly influenced by his intention. Pressure intensity and movement direction do not in this case appear so significant as intention, but they must nevertheless accord with the polarity required.

A tense, spastic, or painful area will be 'drained' by slower and more prolonged movement than the sudden, deeper and more rapid movements used to supplement.

The variant of this, namely use of knuckles and elbow for pressure and movement is merely an application of the same principles but adapted to an appropriate area. We have found massage with the knuckled or the end of the first phalange of index or middle finger to be especially effective on the Gall Meridian points in the vicinity of the head of the great trochanter.

Percussion Massage

Percussion massage will be familiar to anyone who has studied Japanese KUATSU or resuscitation technique. This is not really a suitable technique for clinical practice, but it is admirably suited to emergencies. A practitioner should know something of the technique of percussion.

One, two, or three (*rarely* more than three) short sharp blows are given on the acupuncture point using the end of the first phalange of the index or middle finger. The fist is held closed and with the operating finger or phalange in line with the metacarpal. The range of movement in delivering the percussive blow must not exceed four inches. The heel of the hand is used percussively for an area such as the solar plexis; the knee for mid-dorsal vertebral points; toes for the lowest vertebral points.

The Japanese have developed a highly effective use of SOUND WAVES, involving a peculiar sudden shout or cry, known as KIAI. The KIAI in minor keys, flats and discords produces syncope and paralysis by a nerve re-action which lowers arterial pressure, retards cardiac rhythm and influences certain secretions. The KIAI in major keys, sharps and harmony, of sufficient suddenness and intensity induces excitation and acceleration of respiratory and cardiac function.

10.

Diet

DIET & THE FIVE ELEMENTS. Traditionally the diet has always been considered to have very great therapeutic significance indeed. Not only is it at times possible to treat a condition by diet alone, it is also considered that almost any other method of treatment can be nullified by a continued wrong (inappropriate) diet.

According to the NEI CHING, each Element creates a particular flavour, which *enters* a particular organ, *strengthens and nourishes* an organ, and is *proper food for* a particular organ. Each Flavour has a special POWER, influence or effect: each Flavour, if in excess, is counteracted by one and counteracts another. This may best be appreciated if set out in tabular form.

THE ELEMENTS	WOOD	FIRE	EARTH	METAL	WATER
create the flavours	Sour	Bitter	Sweet	Hot Pungent Aromatic	Salty
which ENTER	Liver	Heart	Spleen	Lungs	Kidneys
STRENGTHEN & NOURISH the	Liver	Heart	Stomach	Lungs	Kidneys
are PROPER FOOD for the	Heart	Lungs	Liver	Kidneys	Spleen
The POWER of the Flavours are	ASTRINGENT GATHERING	DRYING STRENGTHENING	HARMONIZING RETARDING	DISPERSING	SOFTENING

AN EXCESS in the diet of	SOUR	BITTER	SWEET	PUNGENT	SALTY
is COUNTER-ACTED by	PUNGENT	SALTY	SOUR	BITTER	SWEET
and COUNTERACTS	SWEET	PUNGENT	SALTY	SOUR	BITTER

In the NEI CHING we read a great deal about the detrimental effects of the flavours if one flavour exceeds all others in the diet. The items we now give are from the NEI CHING:

EXCESS SOUR Toughens the flesh, is injurious to the muscles, the flesh hardens and wrinkles, the lips become slack, causes the liver to produce excess saliva, and the force of the Spleen will be cut short.

EXCESS BITTER causes Spleen energy to become dry, and Stomach energy becomes dense, congested; withers the skin; body hair falls out.
When there is a disease of the BONES one should not eat too much bitter.

EXCESS SWEET causes aches in the bones; Heart energy will be full, Kidneys will be unbalanced, Hair on the head will fall out.

EXCESS PUNGENT knots the muscles, Muscles and pulses slacken, The Spirit will be injured; Finger and toe nails wither and decay.
When there is an illness of the respiratory tract do not use too much pungent food.

EXCESS SALTY The great bones become weary, muscles and flesh become deficient, the mind becomes despondent; hardens the pulse, tears appear, complexion changes.
When there is a disease of the blood do not use too much salty food.

We now give a few indications from the NEI CHING regarding when to prescribe or use the various flavours. The quaint terminology of the NEI CHING is retained.

SOUR: Sour food has an astringent or gathering effect; thus the HEART suffering from tardiness means that it is devoid of strength, one should eat sour food which has an astringent effect.

In connection with the LIVER, one uses sour food in order to drain and expel.

Sick LUNGS have a tendency to close and to bind, eat sour food in order to make them receive what is due to them. Use sour food to supplement and strengthen the LUNGS.

BITTER: When the SPLEEN suffers from moisture one should eat bitter food which has a drying effect.

When the LUNGS suffer an obstruction of the upper respiratory tract eat bitter food which will disperse the obstruction and restore the flow.

One uses bitter food to drain the SPLEEN.

SWEET: When the LIVER suffers from an acute attack it indicates that there is an excessive fullness of the LIVER; one should quickly eat sweet food to calm it down.

One uses sweet food in order to drain and dispel in connection with the HEART.

A sick SPLEEN has the tendency to work tardily and lazily; then one should eat sweet food to set it at ease, i.e., supplement and strengthen it.

PUNGENT: Use pungent food to drain the LUNGS and make them expel.

When the KIDNEYS suffer from dryness eat pungent food which will moisten them.

Pungent food opens the pores and will bring about free circulation of saliva and fluid secretions.

If the LIVER has the tendency to disintegrate, eat pungent food to supplement the LIVER FUNCTION and to stop leaks.

SALTY: Eat salty food to make the HEART pliable (N.B. use SEA SALT and *not* common salt), to supplement and strengthen the heart.

Eat salty food to drain the KIDNEYS and make them expel.

Acupuncture Never Fails

In one of his books Dr. Nyoiti Sakurazawa makes what, at first sight, appears to be a somewhat arrogant remark. He says that acupuncture never fails, and if after treatment the patient does not get well or has a relapse, it is not the fault of acupuncture but the patient is wrong. A very similar remark was made by the great Samuel Hahnemann as regards homoeopathy. He says that if, after the correct dosage of the simillimum has been given to the patient, the patient does not get well or has a relapse then *it is a sure sign* that there is some external circumstance or habit that is keeping the diseased condition alive, and a cure is not to be expected until and unless that circumstance is altered. This is indeed very true in relation to acupuncture treatment. We assume, of course, that the points have been correctly selected, located and treated.

Among the most important of all external circumstances and habits that militate against complete cure is faulty diet.

After many years of research and experimentation with many different diets (personally tried) we have come to the conclusion that the basics of diet are few and simple.

Consume no more than is sufficient for health.

Too many people eat too much too often. This is not necessarily due to greed or self-indulgence. The body requires certain ingredients in proper quantity, quality and relative proportions. If one or more of these required ingredients has been removed from the food, by refining, the body remains in a permanent state of hunger for that ingredient, and will therefore go on eating (long after the stomach and all other organs complain) in a desperate attempt to find that missing ingredient. Thus, in order to get what is missing, the body will take in an appalling excess of other ingredients which, in proper proportion, would be correct for health but in excess become a killing factor.

Masticate

Food should be chewed until it almost disappears without the need to swallow. The medicine-philosophic reason for this is that matter cannot be integrated, absorbed and made part of a new organism until it has become completely de-polarized. The de-polarization is effected by breaking up the aliments into very small particles all of which must come into contact with the de-polarizing factor, saliva. Every particle of food that is swallowed without being de-polarized acts as an active or potential disruptive disturbing factor.

Items that must be eliminated from the diet

COMMON SALT. This is not easy when one considers that common salt is included in so much tinned, preserved, and packeted foods. Common salt is a killer. Use SEA SALT. Sea salt will never provoke excessive thirst nor cause the many distressing symptoms that follow on common salt intake.

WHITE SUGAR. Cane or beet sugar in the refined white state is to be cut right out of the diet. This again means steering clear of a wide range of tinned and preserved foods.

The coarse brown unrefined muscavado sugar is permitted in moderation. If sweetening is required it is best to use honey in moderation.

WHITE FLOUR & ALL REFINED CEREALS. Grain, the natural food for man, should form 80 per cent, by weight, of his diet, but it must be UNrefined whole grain or whole-flour.

Drastically cut down liquid intake

Urination should not exceed four times per day. This is the best guide as to the correctness of fluid intake. The daily health 'barometer' is the stools. In good health these should be: Long, soft, formed, floating, golden brown, and without unpleasant odour.

Live simply

Living should be a joy, together with all the activities of life.

11.

Psychological Considerations

According to Far-Oriental medicine-philosophy it is accepted as axiomatic that one cannot split mind from body; and one cannot therefore treat the one without affecting the other. The patient is always to be considered as an organism-as-a-whole-in-environments. Environmental factors cannot be separated from a patient. In other words a patient with nothing surrounding him is an absurdity. Therefore the medicine-philosopher teaches that treatment is always to be given with a 'wholeness' orientation.

In the West, in general, there is no medicine-philosophy in the Far-Eastern sense; and one finds 'departmentalisation' with consequent attempts to treat the physical body, or even isolated parts of it, as if the treatment would have no effect upon the rest of the organism. Here and there one does come across medical men who think along lines in conformity with the facts of nature.

The medicine philosophy of Samuel Hahnemann, as expounded in *Organon*, represents the nearest Western medicine philosophy to that of the Far East that we have so far come across. Many passages in this book of his could as easily be imagined as quotations from some Far-Eastern text. The suitability of a 'marriage' between acupuncture and homoeopathy was envisaged by Dr de la Fuÿe, who made what was probably the first attempt to bring these two therapies together. There remains a great deal of research work to be carried out in these two fields.

It is clear, too, that Groddeck thoroughly understood

the inseparable relationships of body-mind; his contri-
butions to the literature of psycho-analysis are world-
renowned. A careful study of Groddeck will bring a
practitioner near to a valid and sound knowledge of what
physical symptoms are to be treated for certain related
mental and emotional disorders and, vice-versa, how to
approach psycho-logically and treat analytically related
physical conditions.

It has been sufficiently demonstrated experimentally for
it to be accepted as an indisputable fact of observation
that: All thought processes and mental states *co-exist* with
related muscular activity and tension. If a therapist is able
to affect muscle tensions and activities he will, *ipso facto*,
affect to the same degree the thought processes and mental
states.

Mental States Responsive to Acupuncture

As regards the treatment of psycho-logical disturbances by
acupuncture, and what mental conditions are likely to
respond to acupuncture, de la Fuÿe makes it quite clear in
his *Treatise*, that mental cases arising out of cerebral
lesions and tissue degeneration are, for the greater part,
not treatable by acupuncture: but the mentally backward,
misfits, mal-adjusted, neurotics (particularly cases of
anxiety neuroses), depressional cases, etc., respond well to
the needles (moxa or massage). He is careful to add that
there are also cases which respond to acupuncture: by
'suggestion'.

Doctor de la Fuÿe emphasizes, and we re-iterate and
emphasize this also, that a practitioner must be supple in
his outlook and not seek at all costs to make any one
method triumph over all others. Above everything else the
practitioner must have the desire to heal the patient: and,
he says, it would be evidence of narrow-mindedness to
reject *a priori* a synthesis of acupuncture and other

methods on the grounds that such a synthesis of methods is not in strict accord with the ancient tradition of 'pure' acupuncture.

The ideal therapist is one whose spirit is pliable enough, and whose knowledge is broad enough for him to use at one and the same time the quintessence of all known reputable methods. There is no need for conflict between adherents of different acupuncture schools, or different methods: on the contrary, the ideal is a combining of them all into the one and only valid therapy — the one that heals.

As far as we have been able to understand Far-Eastern medicine-philosophy the Far-Eastern practitioner *never* relied upon acupuncture as the sole means of effecting a cure. It was always accompanied by some other supporting treatment according to the patient's needs — be it by diet, exercise, baths, manipulations, herbal remedies, lotions, liniments, potions, packs, plasters, poultices, etc.

When we talk about treatment of the psyche we are not thinking in terms of modern Western psychiatry, with use of shock and drugs, but rather in terms of psycho-analysis and systems derived therefrom.

Anyone who has been through the two years psycho-analysis considered in some quarters as the necessary qualification to practise analysis (that is to say not less than two hundred hours of analysis spread over two years) will be only too painfully aware that:

(a) Psycho-analysis, from the patient's point of view, can be an expensive way of having the psyche treated; especially as a beneficial outcome is by no means certain.

(b) Whether it is in the end successful or not, psycho-analysis seems inevitably to be accompanied by a great deal of emotional torment and distress.

Acupuncture Linked with Psycho-Analysis
It is desirable, therefore, that there should be some

alternative and far speedier method of resolving analytical problems. But this does not mean to say that we regard Chinese acupuncture by itself as an alternative to psycho-analysis in all cases; but rather do we intend to convey that a judicious use of Chinese acupuncture points can serve as an extremely useful technique for bringing about more rapid results, without torment, and with greater predict-ability.

If one wants classical justification for linking psycho-analysis with acupuncture, we draw attention to the passages in the NEI CHING dealing with interpretation of dreams. Several thousand years before Freud the Chinese recognized that dreams represent a mechanism for symbolic wish-fulfilment.

There should be no difficulty in appreciating that any disturbances in the flow and balance of Life-Force, with its two poles YANG and YIN, manifests itself as a disturbance of some degree in both psyche and soma.

In our own analytical experience and practise of physiotherapy and acupuncture we have found confirm-ation of Groddeck's findings, and we feel that it is beyond dispute that an habitual state of mind sooner or later will shew itself in analagous or related states of body.

YIN and YANG Fears

As an example: FEAR, whether acute or chronic, is suitably labelled a 'state of mind'. Fear has also its physical manifestations. Fear does not always manifest physically in the same way. We can divide the fear manifestations into two broad categories, YIN or YANG.

In the one type, YIN, the person goes *limp* with fear; rooted to the spot out of a feeling of utter weakness and inability to act. There is an urge to flight, but no power to do so. Muscles seem paralysed — there may be inconti-nence through vesical paresis — there may be diarrhoea, etc.

When treating a patient shewing a psycho-logical state of fear of this kind, one works on the basis that *if* any physical disturbances happen they will be of the kind just listed; and even if these physical symptoms are absent, an acupuncture point or points is selected at which these symptoms would be treated should they actually occur. YIN fear would therefore be treated as for urine incontinence through vesical paresis, and/or diarrhoea, and/or extreme weakness, etc. Fear of this kind reflects a depletion of vital energy, deficiency on the heart, etc. One might even treat as for paralysis of the muscles of the larynx (the patient wants to cry out but is unable to make a sound).

In the other type of fear, YANG, instead of making the subject limp with fear, it makes him *stiff* with fear. Instead of the urge to flight, there is the urge to fight, but an aggressive urge accompanied by indecision. Physical symptoms, if present, would include incontinence; but this time due to vesical spasm. The urge to aggressive action tenses the muscles. A point or points would be chosen *as if* the appropriate physical symptoms were actually present and, to some degree, they certainly will be. One treates as for cramp, spasm, convulsions even; and selects points such as 'the anticonvulsive: II.3 (the Wood point of the Small Intestine) or VIII.3 (The Earth point of the Liver, an anti-cramp point) or VII.34 (Earth point of the Gall) or VII.40 (the Organ point of the Gall) and so on.

Anger, a child of fear, is from an analytical viewpoint often treated as an aggressive manifestation of fear. According to Groddeck and others (confirmed in our own experience) suppressed anger leads to *chronic* tenseness in arm and shoulder musculature; to neuritis pains in the arms, and so on. One of the acupuncture points at which these physical symptoms is treated is V.9 (the Wood point of the Circulation).

Popular expressions often give valuable clues to a psychological state. For example, when referring to a circumstance that makes him angry a person exclaims, 'How galling'. This would at once turn our minds to the Gall Bladder meridian where one would expect to find a disturbance of excess or congestion.

Fixed Ideas Precede Stiff Joints

Rigidities on the level of the psyche will tend to externalize corresponding rigidities on the level of the soma. Fixed ideas are all too often the precursors of fixed or stiff joints. Even if articular or muscular rigidities are not yet present one would select points to treat as if they were. Rigid narrow minds, obstinacy and stubbornness that refuses to re-evaluate prejudices, etc., would be treated as for arthritis, muscular rheumatism, fibrositis, etc. The pulses would, of course, be consulted for confirmation.

Many worries, anxieties, power-complexes, and sexual problems are linked with constipations, haemorrhoids, ear, nose, and throat troubles.

There is another point generally overlooked by the practitioner: and this applies to ANY form of therapy. One does come across the rare instance when the practitioner is confident that a correct diagnosis has been made, and an equally correct treatment given – but the patient responds in the opposite way to that expected. The therapist should always be prepared for the stimulus of the symbolism in the treatment evoking a reaction in the psyche which is the polar opposite of the expected physical reaction to the physical stimulus. It does occasionally happen that the stimulus of the symbol overpowers the physical stimulus sufficiently to aggravate a polar opposite reaction.

12.

The Five Emotions

It is our carefully considered opinion that for the treatment of psycho-logical disturbances we have, in acupuncture, one of the most powerful of all therapy methods so far discovered by man. For the practitioner whose interest is principally upon the psychological approach we recommend a serious consideration of the FIVE ELEMENTS arrangement of Emotions, together with the Generation and the Control cycles. The FIVE primary emotions or urges are these: FEAR, ANGER, JOY, SYMPATHY, GRIEF. These we shall now briefly discuss.

According to NEI CHING each pair of organ meridians' energies and the appropriate Element is associated with certain emotions, abilities, capacities, activities, etc. The Primary Emotions we have listed are those given in Ilsa Veith's translation of the NEI CHING. With all due respect to the scholarly work of Ilsa Veith, we are not satisfied that these words cover what is traditionally meant. The Chinese written language uses a symbol to convey an idea practically impossible to translate by one word only: and, generally speaking, it would be far too cumbersome to use a whole sentence (or more) each time one wished to refer to an emotion. It is expedient to continue using Ilsa Veith's translation, but first to explain something of what we understand is to be included in the 'idea'.

Joy

As a basic or primary emotion, Joy is said to arise out of the activity of the divinely inspired part of man. Four organs are linked with this emotion: Heart, Circulation, Small Intestine, and Three-Heater. Joy represents the feeling of *Inspiration and versatility of the Spiritual (psychic) faculties* which becomes possible to living creatures only when the human stage has been reached, with the symbol forming an interpretative faculty. The associated sense, often translated as *Speech Sense*, includes all that can come under the heading *Communication Sense*. This of course includes all communication by means of symbol and and is not restricted to verbal language.

One of the highest expressions of well-balanced Joy is laughter. Here naturally we mean laughter as a healthy expression of organismic well-being and happiness.

An imbalance in the energies of Heart, Small Intestine, Circulation and Three-Heater (I, II, V, & VI) will have various effects. In Excess there may be Euphoria and/or certain manifestations of Hysteria, for example. This could be accompanied by a pulse indication of Excess on the Heart meridian (I) requiring dispersion. An acupuncture point traditionally indicated for the treatment of hysteria is the fourth point of the Heart (I.4); this is the Metal point on the Heart meridian.

An insufficiency of Joy is indicated by Sadness, this is not the same as Grief. Grief is a positive emotion, whereas Sadness is a negative emotion of 'insufficiency'. There are two points of especial significance here. The imbalance giving rise to insufficient *joie de vivre* may be due to a deficiency of Fire, shewn on the Heart pulse as a deficiency, coupled with a possible excess on the Earth organs. In this case the indicated point for treatment is the Earth point of the Heart meridian which is also the Source or Organ point of the Heart, point number seven.

This point has been appropriately nicknamed by de la Fuÿe '*Joie de Vivre*'. Clinical use of this point in stimulation has confirmed its efficacy for mental depression, sadness, etc. The other point of special interest likely to be indicated is I.5, the Passage point on the Heart meridian from the Small Intestine meridian. This point is indicated if the imbalance is on the Fire Element itself; that is to say, an imbalance between the various Fire Element organs, when the Excess shews on the Alimentary and the Deficiency on the Distributive organs.

An insufficiency or breakdown in communication may express itself as Deafness to the Human voice: this is treatable at, for example, VI.10, V.7 & .9 as well as local points on the Small Intestine and Three-Heater meridians.

On the *Generation Cycle* Joy is the Mother of Sympathy: and on the *Control Cycle* Joy counteracts Grief and is counteracted by Fear.

Sympathy

As a basic emotion Sympathy represents the feeling of 'including environment as part of one's self' or taking in the extraneous and making it one's own. Here Sympathy represents broad appreciation and understanding that results from healthy well-balanced *Ideas*, focused *Thoughts*, calm and collected *Thinking*. In another terminology Sympathy stands for the *Caritas aspect of Love*, the enfolding, including aspect. This emotion is linked with the Earth Organs, Stomach and Spleen. It is also linked with TASTE and Discrimination: the selection of what is to be included in self and what is not to be so included.

On the *Control Cycle* Sympathy counteracts Fear and is counteracted by Anger. On the *Generation Cycle* Sympathy engenders Grief.

Grief

We differentiate Sadness from Grief or Sorrow. Sadness is simply an absence of Joy, whereas Grief is considered a positive emotion in its own right. This is the emotion felt upon parting. According to tradition it belongs to the organs associated with elimination, and with what the Chinese call the 'inferior animal spirit', Lungs and Large Intestine.

In proper balance this is a healthy emotion and a very necessary awareness of 'when to let go' and 'when something has been taken away'. In times of stress this gives rise to the ability to weep and to wail.

Even in Western psycho-logical circles it is well recognized that grief (awareness of loss and elimination) is linked with Lung function. Various power complexes, parsimony, unwillingness to experience loss, etc., are linked with large Intestine functioning causing Constipations and so on. Mental depressions are often treated at X.4 to stimulate elimination of toxic thought; and Mental confusion and depression may be treated at X.11.

On the *Control Cycle* Grief is counteracted by Joy, and counteracts Anger. On the *Generation Cycle* a healthy sense of awareness of Loss engenders a healthy sense of values, resulting in AWE, Reverence, or Fear.

Fear

In this one term, Fear, are to be included the notions of Awe, Reverence and Wonder as well as Timidity. A healthy Fear is an awareness of one's limitations of ability, strength, circumstance, etc., and of Relativity generally. This emotion belongs to the Element with which are associated Will and Resolution; the aspect concerned with calling to Life that which is dormant, and with death.

As a healthy emotion it enables one to recognize danger and, in the face of danger, to react appropriately. This is associated with the energies corresponding to the Water Element organs, Bladder and Kidneys.

Courage is not the opposite of Fear in the sense of indicating an *absence* or deficiency of Fear; but rather Courage indicates a *healthy* Fear or awareness of danger, risks, hazards, etc., together with a well-balanced Will and Resolution. Courage also indicates a strong Fire or Self-confidence. Deficiency on the Water Element would lead to Foolhardiness, not Courageous action.

On the *Control Cycle* Fear counteracts Joy, and is counteracted by Sympathy. This may be illustrated, for example in the instance of excessive Awe/Wonder amounting to superstitious Fear being counteracted by an adequate awareness of what may properly be included as part of one's self or within one's own control. The Kidneys are organs of Filtration and as such (the general secernent organ of the whole body) belong appropriately to the function of both Calling to Life and to Bringing to an end.

On the *Generation cycle*, Fear is said to be the mother of Anger.

Anger
We had difficulty in finding a suitable term to replace Anger, which tends, in the West to have derogatory implications. Traditionally Anger is the emotion of the Soul or Spiritual faculties in self-urge or birth and growth of the Ego. This represents the healthy urge to become something, to live, to expand, combating restrictive environment much as a plant pushes itself upwards through the soil towards light or the germinating seed splits the husk apart, or a chick breaks through the shell. This urge could as suitably be called *Aggression*. This is a necessary urge which, well-balanced, is conducive to health.

In this sense it becomes clear how 'Anger' can be the mother of Joy, as on the *Generation Cycle* Wood is the mother of Fire. Only an adequate self-expansion and growth can engender awareness of maturity, strength, self-confidence and so on which all together constitute Joy. On the *Control Cycle* Anger is subdued by Grief, and counteracts Sympathy.

It will have been noticed that 'Love' is not looked upon as a simple or primary emotion. What we in the West include under the one label 'Love' has, in Far-Oriental thought, at least two components.

The positive aspect or 'Eros' is a self-striving of self for self. Eros can be cruel, as even on occasions it must properly be, in upward thrusting of self. Eros is an 'exclusive' emotion.

Love has however its other pole, the 'inclusive', 'enfolding', 'receiving', or making and accepting as one with one's self. This is the 'Caritas' aspect. Caritas is equated with Sympathy.

The organs traditionally associated with Anger are Liver and Gall, and belong to the Wood Element.

In the Christian Scriptural text 'Perfect Love casteth out Fear' we have a Western re-statement of the Far-Oriental doctrine 'Perfected or *completed* Love, namely the Caritas pole Sympathy, counteracts Fear.' This is a simple instance of Natural Control Cycle sequence; or statement of a Law of Nature.

Deep reflection upon the Generation and Control Cycle ordering will reveal the goal towards which the Cosmos is striving, namely, to bring forth in mature fulness the divinely inspired self-conscious awareness in creative communion. This becomes possible for the first time in the evolution of the Cosmos with the appearance of the Human class of life.

Appendix

This Creation Sequence has been compiled from the study of four main sources: (a) The various works of Nyoti Sakurazawa, and his observations on the 'Logarithmic Spiral' (b) Krazinski's *Tibetan Medicine Philosophy* (c) Lorenz OKen's *Elements of Physiophilosophy* and (d) the *Primary Physics* of C.W. Dawson.

It is offered for reflective and speculative thought. It represents our attempt to make preliminary steps in bringing together material from doctrines widely separated in time and space but which seem to have a basic wisdom in common. It also appears to support Korzybski's assertion that man is not an animal, but belongs to a different class of life which he calls 'time-binders'.

COSMOGENY

CREATION SEQUENCE FROM ZERO

1. The Process of Analysis

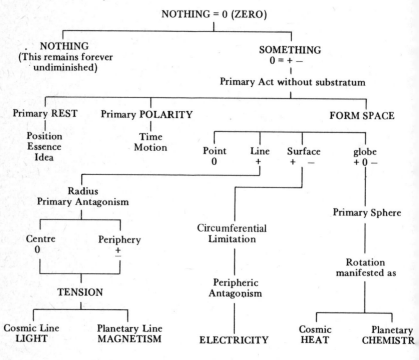

THREE PRIMAL FORMS OF THE WORLD

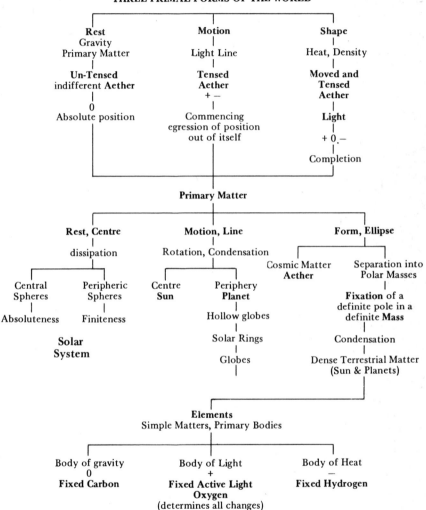

Rest
Gravity
Primary Matter

Un-Tensed
indifferent Aether

0
Absolute position

Motion
Light Line

Tensed
Aether
+ −

Commencing
egression of position
out of itself

Shape
Heat, Density

Moved and
Tensed
Aether

Light

+ 0 −

Completion

Primary Matter

Rest, Centre
dissipation

Central   Peripheric
Spheres   Spheres

Absoluteness   Finiteness

Solar
System

Motion, Line
Rotation, Condensation

Centre   Periphery
Sun   **Planet**

Hollow globes

Solar Rings

Globes

Form, Ellipse

Cosmic Matter   Separation into
Aether   Polar Masses

Fixation of a
definite pole in a
definite **Mass**

Condensation

Dense Terrestrial Matter
(Sun & Planets)

Elements
Simple Matters, Primary Bodies

Body of gravity   Body of Light   Body of Heat
0   +   −
Fixed Carbon   **Fixed Active Light**   **Fixed Hydrogen**
                         Oxygen
                         (determines all changes)

FIRST GENERAL MATTERS (ELEMENTS)

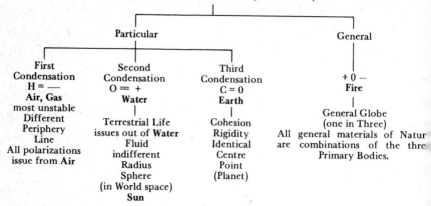

Particular

First Condensation
H = —
Air, Gas
most unstable
Different
Periphery
Line
All polarizations
issue from **Air**

Second Condensation
O = +
Water

Terrestrial Life
issues out of **Water**
Fluid
indifferent
Radius
Sphere
(in World space)
Sun

Third Condensation
C = 0
Earth

Cohesion
Rigidity
Identical
Centre
Point
(Planet)

General

+ 0 —
Fire

General Globe
(one in Three)
All general materials of Nature
are combinations of the three
Primary Bodies.

FUNCTIONS OF THE GENERAL ELEMENTS

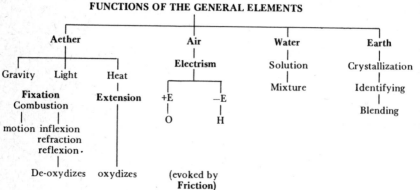

Aether

Gravity   Light   Heat

Fixation
Combustion
|
motion inflexion
refraction
reflexion·

Extension

De-oxydizes   oxydizes

Air

Electrism

+E   —E
| |
O   H

(evoked by
Friction)

Water

Solution
|
Mixture

Earth

Crystallization
|
Identifying
|
Blending

Here the Process of Analysis ends
and the Process of Synthesis Begins

THE FIVE KINGDOMS OF NATURE

Inorganic	Organic Moved			Psychic Motive
Quiescent				
Non-Moving	Internally	Sexually	Throughout	(Symbol forming)
(1) Minerals	(2) Plants	(3) Sex	(4) Animals	(5) Humans
Parts of a plant	Whole planet	Solar?	Sun & Planet	micro-cosmos
	Bound in Space	Transitory	Free-Movement in Space	Free-Movement in Time Symbolism Reasoning
Chemical	Galvanic (Electro-chemical)	Sentient	nervose mobile	
changes proceed from external circumstances	a Chemical power constantly excited by electrism		Galvanic and Sentient	chemico - galvano Sentient self-conscious ratiocinative (free comparison)
(no New Tensions can originate)	(Constant Re-Newal of tension)		Mental functions without ratiocination	
Magnetism & Chemism	self-excitation of the individualizing element			
"Earth" (Chi of **Badgan**)	"Metal" (Badgan-	"Water" Schara	"Wood" Chi-	"Fire" (Badgan of **Chi**)

of
Schara

Bibliography

HUANG TI NEI CHING SU WEN, trans. Ilza Veith, Baltimore 1949.
I CHING, 2 Vols. Routledge & Kegan Paul, 1951.
TAO TEH CHING, trans. Arthur Waley, G. Allen & Unwin, 1934.
The Secret of the Golden Flower, Routledge & Kegan Paul, 1950.
Formulaire D'Acupuncture, WU WEI PING, Lib. Maloine Paris, 1959.
Principe Unique, Nyoiti Sakurazawa, J. Vrin, Paris, 1958.
La Philosophie de la Médecine d'Extrême-Orient, Nyoti Sakurazawa, J. Vrin, Paris, 1959.
Traité d'Acupuncture, Roger de la Fuÿe, Paris, 1956.
Cours du Docteur de la Fuÿe, Societe Française d'Acupuncture.
Akupunktur als Neuraltherapie, Erich W. Stiefvater, Haug, 1956.
Die Tiebetische Medizinphilosophie P. Cyrill von Korvin-Krasinski, Origo Verlag, 1953.
Tibetische Heilkumde, Theodor Burang, Origo Verlag, 1957.
Das Buch vom Ess, Georg Groddeck, Vienna, 1926.
Elements of Physiophilosophy, Lorenz Oken, London, 1847.
Physics of the Primary State of Matter, Cyril W. Davson, London, 1955.
The Mysterious Universe, James Jeans, F.R.S., 1930.
An Introduction to Symbolic Logic, Suzanne K. Langer, New York, 1953.
Progressive Relaxation, Edmund Jacobson, Chicago, 1938.
Science & Sanity, Alfred Korzybski, Institute of General Semantics, 1948 3rd Edition.
Scientific Epistemologic Backgrounds of General Semantics, Marjorie A. Swanson, I.G.S., 1959.
Organon of Medicine, Samuel Hahnemann, Boericke & Tafel, 1952.
The Science of Tridosha, Dr. B. Bhattacharya, New York, 1956.

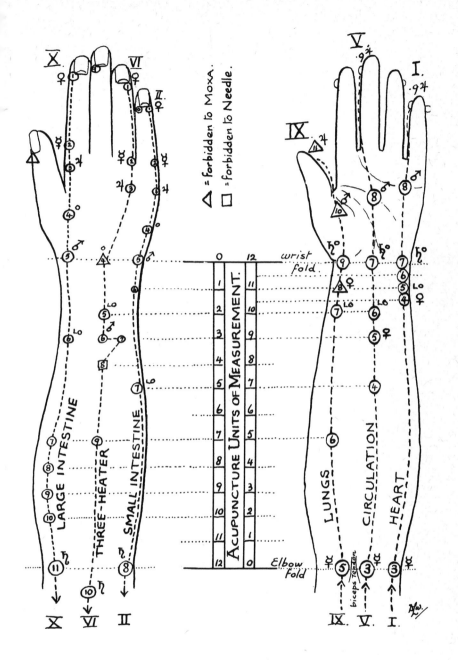

△ = forbidden to Moxa.
□ = forbidden to Needle.

X LARGE INTESTINE
VI THREE-HEATER
II SMALL INTESTINE

ACUPUNCTURE UNITS OF MEASUREMENT.

0	12
1	11
2	10
3	9
4	8
5	7
6	6
7	5
8	4
9	3
10	2
11	1
12	0

wrist fold

Elbow Fold

biceps tendon

LUNGS CIRCULATION HEART

IX V I

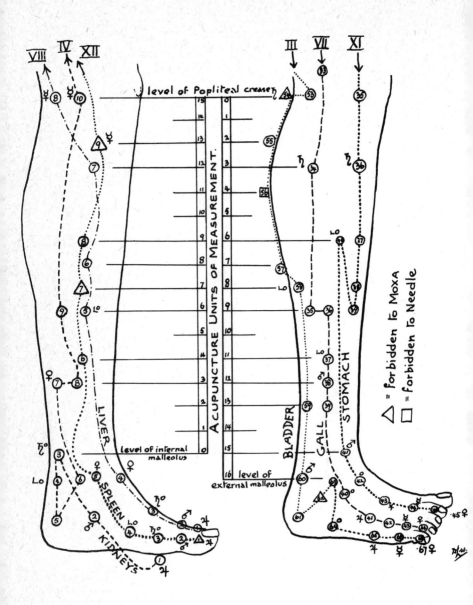

level of Popliteal crease

ACUPUNCTURE UNITS OF MEASUREMENT.

level of internal malleolus

level of external malleolus

LIVER

SPLEEN

KIDNEYS

BLADDER

GALL

STOMACH

△ = forbidden to Moxa

☐ = forbidden to Needle

VIII   IV   XII

III   VII   XI